# A Practical Guidebook in
# Femoral Neck Fixation System

AF096573

# A Practical Guidebook in
# Femoral Neck Fixation System

### Editor
**Sachin Yashwant Kale**
MS(Orthopedics) D Ortho FCPS Fellowship in Arthroplasty
Professor and Head of Unit
Department of Orthopedics
Dr DY Patil School of Medicine
Navi Mumbai, Maharashtra, India

### Co-Editors

**Arvind J Vatkar**
MS(Orthopedics) AFIH MCh Spine Surgery(Edgehill University,
UK) Advanced Spine Surgery Fellowship(Nottingham UK)
Assistant Professor
Department of Orthopedics
MGM Medical College (Proposed)
Nerul, Navi Mumbai, Maharashtra, India

**Vishal Kumar**
MS DNB FRCS
Professor (Additional)
Department of Orthopedics
PGIMER
Chandigarh, India

### Sub-Editors

**Sanjay Dhar**
MS(Orthopedics) DNB(Orthopedics)
Professor and Head of Unit
Department of Orthopedics
Dr DY Patil School of Medicine
Navi Mumbai, Maharashtra, India

**Ajit Chalak**
MS(Orthopedics)
Associate Professor
Department of Orthopedics
MGM Medical College
Nerul, Navi Mumbai,
Maharashtra, India

**Gaurav Kanade**
MS(Orthopedics) Fellowship in
Arthroplasty
Associate Professor
Department of Orthopedics
Dr DY Patil School of Medicine
Navi Mumbai, Maharashtra, India

**Shivam Mehra**
MBBS MS(Orthopedics) Short-term
Fellowship in Deformity Correction
and Limb Lengthening Surgeries
Consultant, Department of
Orthopedics
Mehra Hospital and Research
Institute
Lucknow, Uttar Pradesh, India

**Nindiya Kapoor Mehra**
BTech Biotechnology(Thapar
University, Patiala) MTech
Biotechnology(IIT Kanpur) Executive
Management Programme in
Entrepreneurship Development
(IIT Delhi) Executive Management
Programme in Hospital
Management(IIM Ahmedabad)
Research Head and
Chief Administrator
Department of Administration
and Research
Mehra Hospital and
Research Institute
Lucknow, Uttar Pradesh, India

**Pramod Bhor**
MS(Orthopedics) MBBS
Director
Department of Orthopedics
Fortis Hiranandani Hospital
Navi Mumbai, Maharashtra, India

**Smruti Sachin Kale**
MBBS DGO
Owner Sachi Hospital
Department of Obstetrician and
Gynecologist
Sachi Hospital Airoli
Navi Mumbai, Maharashtra, India

### Foreword
**Sanjay Dhar**

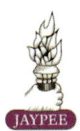

**JAYPEE BROTHERS MEDICAL PUBLISHERS**
*The Health Sciences Publisher*
**New Delhi | London**

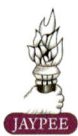 **Jaypee Brothers Medical Publishers (P) Ltd**

**Headquarters**
EMCA House
23/23-B, Ansari Road, Daryaganj
New Delhi 110 002, India
Landline: +91-11-23272143, +91-11-23272703
+91-11-23282021, +91-11-23245672
E-mail: jaypee@jaypeebrothers.com

**Corporate Office**
Jaypee Brothers Medical Publishers (P) Ltd.
4838/24, Ansari Road, Daryaganj
New Delhi 110 002, India
Phone: +91-11-43574357
Fax: +91-11-43574314
E-mail: jaypee@jaypeebrothers.com

**Overseas Office**
JP Medical Ltd.
83, Victoria Street, London
SW1H 0HW (UK)
Phone: +44-20 3170 8910
Fax: +44(0)20 3008 6180
E-mail: info@jpmedpub.com

Website: www.jaypeebrothers.com
Website: www.jaypeedigital.com

© 2025, Jaypee Brothers Medical Publishers

The views and opinions expressed in this book are solely those of the original contributor(s)/author(s) and do not necessarily represent those of editor(s) or publisher of the book.

All rights reserved. No part of this publication may be reproduced, stored or transmitted in any form or by any means, electronic, mechanical, photocopying, recording or otherwise, without the prior permission in writing of the publishers.

All brand names and product names used in this book are trade names, service marks, trademarks or registered trademarks of their respective owners. The publisher is not associated with any product or vendor mentioned in this book.

Medical knowledge and practice change constantly. This book is designed to provide accurate, authoritative information about the subject matter in question. However, readers are advised to check the most current information available on procedures included and check information from the manufacturer of each product to be administered, to verify the recommended dose, formula, method and duration of administration, adverse effects and contraindications. It is the responsibility of the practitioner to take all appropriate safety precautions. Neither the publisher nor the author(s)/editor(s) assume any liability for any injury and/or damage to persons or property arising from or related to use of material in this book.

This book is sold on the understanding that the publisher is not engaged in providing professional medical services. If such advice or services are required, the services of a competent medical professional should be sought.

Every effort has been made where necessary to contact holders of copyright to obtain permission to reproduce copyright material. If any have been inadvertently overlooked, the publisher will be pleased to make the necessary arrangements at the first opportunity.

Inquiries for bulk sales may be solicited at: jaypee@jaypeebrothers.com

*A Practical Guidebook in Femoral Neck Fixation System / Sachin Yashwant Kale*

First Edition: **2025**

ISBN: 978-93-5696-595-9

*Printed at: Sterling Graphics Pvt. Ltd. India*

# Contributors

**Adarsh Tekumalla** MS
Senior Resident
Department of Orthopedics
PGIMER
Chandigarh, India

**Aditya R Gunjotikar** MS(Orthopedics)
Fellowship in Arthroscopy and Sports Medicine
Assistant Professor
Department of Orthopedics
Dr DY Patil School of Medicine
Navi Mumbai, Maharashtra, India

**Aditya Gupta** MS
Senior Resident
Department of Orthopedics
PGIMER
Chandigarh, India

**Ajit Chalak** MS(Orthopedics)
Associate Professor
Department of Orthopedics
MGM Medical College
Nerul, Navi Mumbai, Maharashtra, India

**Ansh Gupta** MS
Senior Resident
Department of Orthopedics
PGIMER
Chandigarh, India

**Arvind J Vatkar** MS(Orthopedics) AFIH
MCh Spine Surgery(Edgehill University, UK) Advanced Spine Surgery Fellowship (Nottingham UK)
Assistant Professor
Department of Orthopedics
MGM Medical College (Proposed)
Nerul, Navi Mumbai, Maharashtra, India

**Gaurav Kanade** MS(Orthopedics)
Fellowship in Arthroplasty
Associate Professor
Department of Orthopedics
Dr DY Patil School of Medicine
Navi Mumbai, Maharashtra, India

**Nindiya Kapoor Mehra** BTech Biotechnology(Thapar University, Patiala) MTech Biotechnology(IIT Kanpur) Executive Management Programme in Entrepreneurship Development(IIT Delhi) Executive Management Programme in Hospital Management(IIM Ahmedabad)
Research Head and Chief Administrator
Department of Administration and Research
Mehra Hospital and Research Institute
Lucknow, Uttar Pradesh, India

**Pramod Bhor** MS(Orthopedics) MBBS
Director
Department of Orthopedics
Fortis Hiranandani Hospital
Navi Mumbai, Maharashtra, India

**Prasad Liladhar Chaudhari** MS DNB D Ortho FCPS Fellowship in Shoulder and Elbow Surgery(ASAN Medical Centre, Seoul, South Korea)
Professor
Department of Orthopedics
Dr DY Patil Medical College and Hospital
Navi Mumbai, Maharashtra, India

**Ronak Mishra** MS(Orthopedics)
Senior Registrar
Department of Orthopedics
Dr DY Patil Hospital and Medical College
Navi Mumbai, Maharashtra, India

## Contributors

**Sachin Yashwant Kale** MS(Orthopedics)
D Ortho FCPS Fellowship in Arthroplasty
Professor and Head of Unit
Department of Orthopedics
Dr DY Patil School of Medicine
Navi Mumbai, Maharashtra, India

**Sandeep N Deore** MS(Orthopedics)
DNB(Orthopedics)
Professor
Department of Orthopedics
Dr DY Patil Medical College
Navi Mumbai, Maharashtra, India

**Sandeep Patel** MS DNB FRCS(Tr & Orth)
Associate Professor
Department of Orthopedics
PGIMER
Chandigarh, India

**Sanjay Dhar** MS(Orthopedics)
DNB(Orthopedics)
Professor and Head of Unit
Department of Orthopedics
Dr DY Patil School of Medicine
Navi Mumbai, Maharashtra, India

**Shikhar D Singh** MS(Orthopedics)
Associate Professor
Department of Orthopedics
Dr DY Patil School of Medicine
Navi Mumbai, Maharashtra, India

**Shivam Mehra** MBBS MS(Orthopedics)
Short-term Fellowship in Deformity
Correction and Limb Lengthening
Surgeries
Consultant
Department of Orthopedics
Mehra Hospital and Research Institute
Lucknow, Uttar Pradesh, India

**Smruti Sachin Kale** MBBS DGO
Owner Sachi Hospital
Department of Obstetrician and
Gynecologist
Sachi Hospital Airoli
Navi Mumbai, Maharashtra, India

**Sunil Shetty** MS(Orthopedics) CCCR
PGDHHM
Professor and Unit Head
Department of Orthopedics
Dr DY Patil School of Medicine
Navi Mumbai, Maharashtra, India

**Sushmit Singh** MBBS MS(Orthopedics)
MRCS
T&O Specialty Registrar
Department of Orthopedics
Warrington and Halton NHS Teaching
Hospitals
Warrington, United Kingdom

**Vaibhav J Koli** MS(Orthopedics)
Fellowship in Arthroscopy and
Arthroplasty
Assistant Professor
Department of Orthopedics
Dr DY Patil Medical College and Hospital
Navi Mumbai, Maharashtra, India

**Vishal Kumar** MS DNB FRCS
Professor (Additional)
Department of Orthopedics
PGIMER
Chandigarh, India

# Foreword

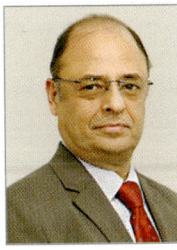

**Sanjay Dhar** MS(Orthopedics) DNB(Orthopedics)
Professor and Head of Unit
Department of Orthopedics
Dr DY Patil School of Medicine
Navi Mumbai, Maharashtra, India

It is with great pleasure that I write the foreword for *"A Practical Guidebook in Femoral Neck Fixation System,"* a comprehensive handbook on the femoral neck system (FNS) for the fixation of femoral neck fractures. This book, expertly edited by Dr Sachin Yashwant Kale, with the collaboration of my esteemed colleagues, Dr Vishal Kumar and Dr Arvind J Vatkar, represents a culmination of years of dedicated research and clinical expertise in the field of orthopedic surgery.

Dr Sachin Yashwant Kale, Professor and Head of Unit in the Department of Orthopedics at Dr DY Patil Medical College and Hospital, Navi Mumbai, Maharashtra, has been a pioneering figure in the study and application of FNS. His vast experience and numerous publications on femoral neck fractures and their complications have made him a leading authority on the subject. Dr Kale's work, including his latest publication on the limitations and complications of FNS, has been instrumental in advancing our understanding and improving patient outcomes in this challenging area of orthopedic surgery.

I have had the privilege of working closely with Dr Sachin Yashwant Kale for many years. Our professional liaison has been marked by numerous collaborative efforts aimed at improving surgical techniques and patient care. His commitment to excellence and innovation is unparalleled, making him exceptionally well suited to edit this handbook.

Dr Vishal Kumar, a Professor at PGIMER, Chandigarh, brings his extensive clinical experience and academic rigor to this work. His notable contributions to the literature on FNS and his role in advancing its application have been widely recognized in the orthopedic community.

Dr Arvind J Vatkar, an orthopedic spine surgeon and Assistant Professor at MGM Medical College, Nerul, Maharashtra, has made significant contributions to the field of orthopedics through his research and publications. He has held various roles, including Senior Spinal Fellow at Queen's Medical Center,

Nottingham University Hospitals, and International Training Fellow at Stepping Hill Hospital. Vatkar's research interests include innovative surgical techniques, fracture management, and advancements in orthopedics and spine surgery.

Dr Sachin Yashwant Kale, Dr Arvind J Vatkar, and Dr Vishal Kumar are experts in the FNS's effectiveness and limits. Dr Kale has conducted substantial study on the clinical efficacy and consequences of FNS, with several publications on the subject. Dr Vatkar has contributed various papers, including a careful comparison of FNS and cannulated compression screws. Dr Kumar has provided vital insights into the use and consequences of FNS in a variety of therapeutic contexts through meta-analysis and clinical experience. Their combined knowledge guarantees that their book gives complete counsel on how to properly use FNS, addressing both its benefits and drawbacks.

This handbook is an essential resource for any orthopedic surgeon seeking to deepen their understanding of femoral neck fracture management using FNS. Dr Kale's leadership in this field, combined with Dr Kumar's and Dr Vatkar's contributions, ensures that this book is both authoritative and practical, providing valuable insights and guidance for improving patient care.

I am confident that readers will find this handbook to be a comprehensive and indispensable guide, reflecting the high standards and innovative approaches that Dr Kale has championed throughout his illustrious career.

# Preface

Femoral neck fractures represent a significant clinical challenge in orthopedics, particularly affecting the young and elderly population and leading to substantial morbidity and healthcare costs. The traditional treatment options, including hemiarthroplasty and various internal fixation techniques, have evolved significantly over the years. Yet, achieving optimal outcomes—balancing effective fracture stabilization with early mobilization and minimal complications—remains a complex endeavor.

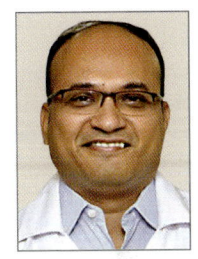

**Sachin Yashwant Kale**

The introduction of the femoral neck system (FNS) in 2017 marked a pivotal advancement in the management of these fractures. The FNS is designed to provide superior stability through its dynamic bolt mechanism, which allows controlled collapse and minimizes the risk of lateral protrusion. This innovation aims to address the limitations of earlier fixation systems, such as the cannulated cancellous screw (CCS) and the dynamic hip screw (DHS), which often required prolonged periods of non-weight bearing, thereby increasing the risk of complications such as pneumonia, deep vein thrombosis, and pressure sores.

This book, *"A Practical Guidebook in Femoral Neck System"*, aims to provide a comprehensive overview of the FNS, detailing its design, biomechanical principles, clinical applications, and rehabilitation protocols. Our objective is to present a thorough examination of the FNS through the lens of current evidence and clinical experience.

The content is structured to guide the reader through various aspects of the FNS:

- *Historical perspective and evolution*: This section outlines the historical development of femoral neck fracture treatments, leading to the advent of the FNS. It includes a discussion on the biomechanical challenges associated with femoral neck fractures and how the FNS addresses these issues.
- *Design and biomechanics*: Detailed descriptions of the FNS design and its biomechanical advantages are presented. This includes comparisons with other fixation systems and a review of relevant biomechanical studies.
- *Clinical applications*: We delve into the practical aspects of using the FNS, from patient selection and surgical techniques to postoperative care. Case studies and clinical trials are discussed to illustrate the efficacy and safety of the FNS in various patient populations.

- *Rehabilitation protocols*: A critical component of the book, this section outlines evidence-based rehabilitation protocols designed to optimize recovery and functional outcomes. Early mobilization strategies, physical therapy exercises, and patient education are thoroughly covered.
- *Outcomes and complications*: This section reviews the clinical outcomes associated with FNS use, including fusion rates, functional scores, and complication rates. Comparative analyses with other fixation methods provide context for understanding the relative benefits and potential risks of the FNS.
- *Future directions*: The final section explores ongoing research, potential advancements, and future directions in the treatment of femoral neck fractures. Emerging technologies and innovations in implant design and rehabilitation are discussed.

Our study, conducted at Dr DY Patil Medical College and Hospital and other hospitals, form a central pillar of this book. It presents a 2-year follow-up of more than 50 patients treated with the FNS, providing valuable insights into the real-world application and outcomes of this system. The data collected includes demographics, fusion rates, functional outcome scores, and complication rates, contributing to a growing body of evidence supporting the FNS.

We hope this book serves as a valuable resource for orthopedic surgeons, researchers, and healthcare professionals involved in the management of femoral neck fractures. By sharing our experience and the broader evidence base, we aim to enhance understanding and improve patient outcomes in this challenging area of orthopedics.

# Preface

Femoral neck fractures are a significant concern, particularly among the young adults, often leading to severe complications and prolonged recovery periods. The introduction of the femoral neck system (FNS) in 2017 has revolutionized the treatment of these fractures. Its minimally invasive design, coupled with a unique dynamic bolt feature, allows for controlled collapse and enhanced fracture stability. This innovation facilitates early mobilization, which is critical for postoperative recovery, reducing the risk of complications and promoting faster rehabilitation.

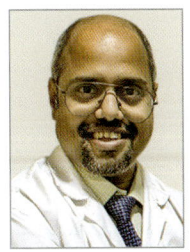

**Arvind J Vatkar**

As editors of this comprehensive guide on the FNS, Dr Sachin Yashwant Kale, Dr Vishal Kumar, and I, Dr Arvind J Vatkar, have dedicated significant effort to ensure that this book serves as an essential resource for orthopedic surgeons and orthopedic resident doctors. Our confidence in writing this book stems from our extensive research and numerous publications on the subject. Dr Vishal Kumar's meta-analysis has provided invaluable insights into the efficacy of the FNS, while Dr Sachin Yashwant Kale and I have extensively studied and documented the complications associated with femoral neck fractures and their treatments.

This book is the culmination of years of hard work, research, and collaboration. We have meticulously compiled the latest data, clinical studies, and expert opinions to provide a thorough understanding of the FNS. We also presented the FNS procedure, including an explanation of the equipment as well as tips and tactics for effective FNS fixation surgery. Hence, it combines more practical and theoretical parts of FNS. It also discusses FNS's complications and reasons behind it, which helps you understand when and how to utilize it effectively, ultimately improving patient outcomes.

We extend our heartfelt gratitude to all the contributing authors whose expertise and dedication have been instrumental in bringing this book to fruition. Each chapter reflects the collective wisdom and experience of leading professionals in the field of orthopedic surgery.

Finally, we would like to thank Jaypee Brothers Medical Publishers for their unwavering support and commitment to disseminating medical knowledge. Their assistance has been invaluable in making this book a reality.

We hope that this book will serve as a valuable reference and inspire continued advancements in the treatment of femoral neck fractures.

# Preface

This compendium is a treatise for the orthopedics and trauma surgeons across the globe. Hip fractures are so common that any orthopedics and trauma surgeon get it in bounty along his clinical practice. This handy handbook is a reference in toto for the femoral neck system (FNS) implant which promises to have a significant advancement in terms of ease and vivid indications of fixation for femoral neck fractures. The authors of the different and diverse chapters covering all the aspects and issues regarding this fracture fixation system are experienced orthopedic trauma surgeons of international accolades, hence marking and making this a tangible reference book for the same. The chapters concerned are illustrious with evidence amalgamated into them from the personal and professional experience of the authors, hence shaping it into a practical book to be used as a guide in day-to-day practices of an orthopedic and trauma surgeon dealing with such fractures. The radiology and the pictures are self-explanatory, thus adding enough wisdom to this must-keep book for any orthopedics and trauma surgeon. This book has chapters including anecdotal notes for the fixation system, pearls and wisdom to use this system flawlessly, and hitherto tackling of complications if otherwise happens in a seamless manner, hence a complete, crisp coterie on FNS implant with charts, figures, and diagrams as special value additions.

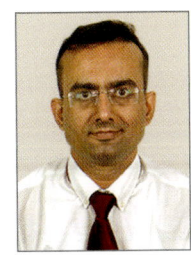

**Vishal Kumar**

Wish you all a happy and meaningful read!

# Acknowledgments

Writing this book has been an extraordinary journey, and I am deeply grateful to all those who have supported and inspired me along the way.

First and foremost, I want to express my heartfelt gratitude to my family—to my spouse, Smruti, whose unwavering support, patience, and encouragement have been my anchor throughout this project and to my daughters, Sachiti and Saanvi, whose curiosity and love have been my constant source of motivation. Your belief in me has made this achievement possible.

I am profoundly thankful to my editors, whose keen insights, meticulous attention to detail, and thoughtful feedback have significantly improved this work. Your guidance and expertise have been invaluable.

I would like to acknowledge my publisher, Jaypee Brothers Medical Publishers, for believing in this book and providing the resources and platform to bring it to life. Your professionalism and commitment have been instrumental in realizing this dream.

I extend my thanks to my friends and colleagues in the medical and academic communities for their contributions, whether through stimulating discussions, providing research support, or offering encouragement.

I am also grateful to the patients who have shared their experiences and insights with me. Their stories have shaped this book and reinforced the importance of our work.

Finally, I want to thank my readers. Their interest and engagement inspire me to continue exploring and sharing knowledge. I hope this book serves as a valuable resource and offers support during the planning.

Thank you all for being part of this journey!

With gratitude,
**Sachin Yashwant Kale**

# Contents

**CHAPTER 1:** **Introduction to Femoral Neck Fractures**      1
*Sachin Yashwant Kale, Arvind J Vatkar, Vaibhav J Koli, Sandeep N Deore, Ronak Mishra*
- Definition and Classification of Femoral Neck Fractures    *1*
- Epidemiology and Incidence Rates, Especially in the Young Population    *3*
- Challenges and Complications Associated with Femoral Neck Fractures    *4*

**CHAPTER 2:** **Anatomy and Biomechanics of the Femoral Neck**      7
*Pramod Bhor, Shivam Mehra, Sushmit Singh, Shikhar D Singh, Sachin Yashwant Kale*
- Detailed Anatomy of the Femoral Neck and Surrounding Structures    *7*
- Biomechanical Principles Relevant to Femoral Neck Fractures and Fixation    *8*
- Understanding Load-bearing Capacity and Stress Distribution in the Femoral Neck    *9*

**CHAPTER 3:** **Evolution of Femoral Neck System Implants**      11
*Sanjay Dhar, Gaurav Kanade, Arvind J Vatkar, Sachin Yashwant Kale*
- Historical Overview of Femoral Neck Fracture Treatment Methods    *11*
- Introduction to the Concept of Modern Implants and their Evolution    *13*
- Comparative Analysis of Various Fixation Methods and their Outcomes    *13*

**CHAPTER 4:** **Design Principles and Components of Femoral Neck System Implants**      15
*Ansh Gupta, Sandeep Patel, Ajit Chalak, Arvind J Vatkar, Sunil Shetty, Vishal Kumar*
- A Summary of the Design Characteristics of Femoral Neck System Implants    *15*

**CHAPTER 5: Preoperative Evaluation and Surgical Planning** .......... 18
*Gaurav Kanade, Sachin Yashwant Kale, Sanjay Dhar, Aditya R Gunjotikar*

- Comprehensive Assessment of Patients with Femoral Neck Fractures  *18*
- Radiological Evaluation Techniques and their Role in Surgical Planning  *19*
- Considerations for Patient-specific Factors and Surgical Approach Selection  *20*

**CHAPTER 6: Step-by-Step Guide to Surgical Procedures for Femoral Neck Fracture Fixation** .......... 22
*Sachin Yashwant Kale, Prasad Liladhar Chaudhari, Arvind J Vatkar, Shikhar D Singh*

- Surgical Approaches, Positioning, and Intraoperative Considerations  *22*

**CHAPTER 7: Postoperative Care and Rehabilitation Protocols** .......... 28
*Shivam Mehra, Nindiya Kapoor Mehra, Pramod Bhor, Aditya R Gunjotikar*

- Immediate Postoperative Management Strategies  *28*
- Rehabilitation Guidelines for Early Mobilization and Functional Recovery  *29*
- Monitoring for Complications and Long-term Follow-up Recommendations  *29*

**CHAPTER 8: Complications and Management Strategies** .......... 31
*Adarsh Tekumalla, Sandeep Patel, Sachin Yashwant Kale, Arvind J Vatkar, Vishal Kumar*

- Overview of Common Complications Associated with Femoral Neck System Implants  *31*
- Identification, Prevention, and Management of Complications During the Perioperative Period  *31*
- Strategies for Salvage Procedures in Case of Implant Failure or Complications  *32*

**CHAPTER 9: Outcomes and Clinical Cases** .......... 37
*Pramod Bhor, Shivam Mehra, Sushmit Singh, Sachin Yashwant Kale, Prasad Liladhar Chaudhari*

- Review of Clinical Outcomes and Functional Results Following Femoral Neck Fracture Fixation  *37*
- Summary of Key Findings From Relevant Clinical Studies and Meta-analyses  *37*
- Discussion on the Evidence-based Approach to Decision-making in Femoral Neck Fracture Management  *38*

CHAPTER 10: **Future Perspectives and Innovations**     47
*Ajit Chalak, Gaurav Kanade, Sachin Yashwant Kale,
Nindiya Kapoor Mehra, Smruti Sachin Kale, Sandeep N Deore*

- Emerging Trends and Advancements in Femoral Neck System Implants    47
- Predictions for the Future Direction of Research and Technology in this Field    47
- Recommendations for Continued Professional Development and Staying Abreast of New Developments    48

CHAPTER 11: **Conclusion: Summary and Key Takeaways**     49
*Sachin Yashwant Kale, Aditya Gupta, Vishal Kumar, Arvind J Vatkar*

**Publications**     53

**Index**     55

# CHAPTER 1

# Introduction to Femoral Neck Fractures

Sachin Yashwant Kale, Arvind J Vatkar, Vaibhav J Koli, Sandeep N Deore, Ronak Mishra

## ■ DEFINITION AND CLASSIFICATION OF FEMORAL NECK FRACTURES

Neck of femur (NOF) fracture is a musculoskeletal injury, caused by an injury in the proximal section of the femur, notably the area where the femoral head connects to the shaft. These fractures are more typically caused by high-energy trauma in younger people or low-energy trauma in elderly people who have low bone density.

Anatomical classification of NOF fractures is based on the site and displacement of the fracture. Fractures may be classified as subcapital, transcervical, or basicervical depending on their location relative to the position of femoral neck and head junction **(Fig. 1A)**. Subcapital fractures occur just below the femoral head, transcervical fractures traverse the neck, and basicervical fractures extend into the upper part of the femoral shaft.

Furthermore, the Garden classification system is often used to characterize the level of displacement in femoral neck fractures. It is divided into four stages: Stage I (incomplete or impacted fracture), stage II (complete fracture with no displacement), stage III (complete fracture and partial displacement), and stage IV (full fracture with entire displacement) **(Fig. 1B)**. Garden classification helps to assess fracture stability and guide surgical care, with higher stages suggesting an increased likelihood of nonunion and avascular necrosis (AVN). Incorporating both Pauwels and Garden classifications enhances the comprehensive evaluation of femoral neck fractures, facilitating tailored treatment approaches and improved patient outcomes.

Pauwels classification is another prominent approach for classifying femoral neck fractures that utilizes the inclination of the fracture line to the horizontal line. Pauwels divided fractures into three distinct groups: Type I (any angle below 30°), type II (30°–50°), and type III (>50°) **(Fig. 1C)**. This categorization method aids in the prediction of fracture stability and informs treatment options, with larger Pauwels' angles linked to increased shear force, thereby leading to an increased risk of displacement and consequences.

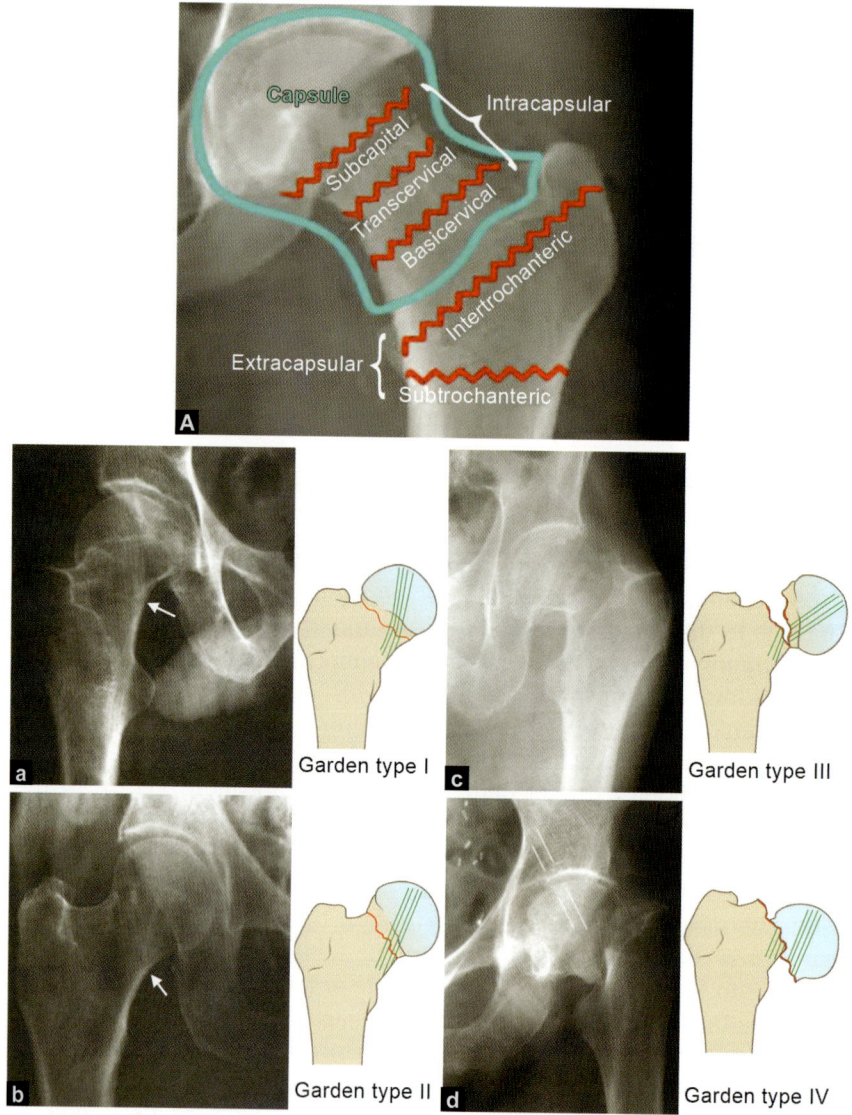

**FIGS. 1A TO C:** *Continued*

*Continued*

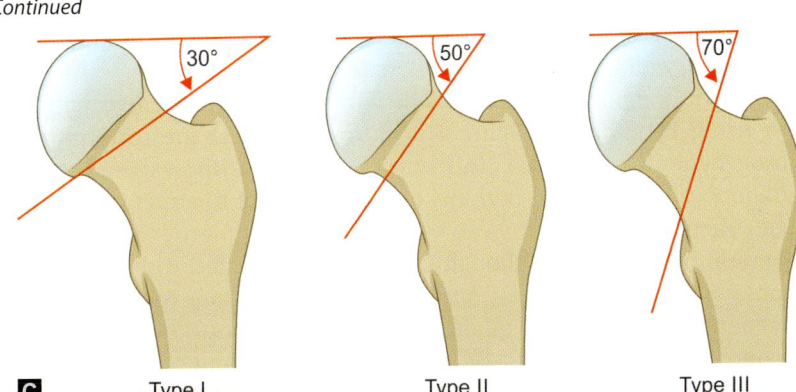

**FIGS. 1A TO C:** Classification of femoral neck fractures: (A) Anatomical classification; (B) Garden classification. The Garden classification of femoral neck fractures: Type I fractures can be incomplete, but much more typically they are impacted into valgus, and retroversion (a). Type II fractures are complete, but undisplaced. These rare fractures have a break in the trabeculations, but no shift in alignment (b). Type III fractures have marked angulation, but usually minimal to no proximal translation of the shaft (c). In the Garden type IV fracture, there is complete displacement between fragments and the shaft translates proximally (d). The head is free to realign itself within the acetabulum, and the primary compressive trabeculae of the head and acetabulum realign (white lines); (C) Pauwels classification. The Pauwels classification of femoral neck fractures is based on the angle the fracture forms with the horizontal plane. As the fracture progresses from type I to III, the obliquity of the fracture line increases and, theoretically, the shear forces at the fracture site also increase.

## Summary

Femoral neck fractures are injuries near the femoral head, categorized by their location as subcapital, transcervical, or basicervical, and by displacement using the Garden or Pauwels classifications. These classifications help to determine fracture stability and guide treatment, with Garden stages assessing displacement and Pauwels' angle indicating shear forces and risk of complications.

## ■ EPIDEMIOLOGY AND INCIDENCE RATES, ESPECIALLY IN THE YOUNG POPULATION

Hip fractures in the elderly are associated with a significant mortality rate, with 1-year mortality estimated to be between 20 and 30%. The yearly incidence of hip fractures in India is expected to be >120 per 100,000 people over the age of 50 years. Hip fractures are predicted to rise in India as the country's senior population grows. Femoral neck fractures have grown increasingly prevalent in younger age-groups as the number of high-velocity accidents and sports injuries has increased. Young adults account for 2–3% of all femoral neck fractures, which are commonly caused by high-intensity trauma. Femoral neck fractures in young people are associated with a greater frequency of osteonecrosis, which can range from 12 to 86%.

The world's aging population will confront the problem of dealing with a rising incidence of femoral neck fractures and the resulting cost strain on healthcare systems. This burden comprises the expenditures of rehabilitation, therapy, and perhaps ongoing medical treatment for people with hip fractures.

Femoral neck fractures, though commonly associated with the elderly, also pose a significant burden on the young population, with substantial implications for morbidity, quality-adjusted life years (QALY) loss, and economic costs globally. According to recent epidemiological studies, femoral neck fractures affect over 1.6 million individuals annually worldwide, with approximately 15–20% occurring in individuals under 65 years old, especially males.

These fractures contribute significantly to morbidity, often resulting in extended hospital stays, functional limitations, and increased risks of complications such as AVN and nonunion. Additionally, femoral neck fractures lead to a considerable loss of QALYs due to decreased mobility, chronic pain, and diminished quality of life. For instance, studies have shown that the QALY loss associated with femoral neck fractures can range from 0.1 to 0.6 per fracture, depending on factors such as age and comorbidities.

From an economic standpoint, femoral neck fractures incur substantial costs, including direct expenses related to medical treatment, surgery, rehabilitation, and long-term care, as well as indirect costs stemming from productivity loss and caregiver burden. The economic cost of NOF fractures is estimated to be in the lakhs of crores per year worldwide, emphasizing the need for efficient preventive measures, prompt treatment, and comprehensive medical regulations to reduce the impact of this debilitating trauma on individuals and healthcare systems around the world.

## Summary

Femoral neck fractures, though often associated with the elderly, are increasingly seen in younger populations due to high-velocity trauma, representing 2–3% of all cases. The incidence is rising globally, leading to significant healthcare costs and impacts on quality of life.

## ■ CHALLENGES AND COMPLICATIONS ASSOCIATED WITH FEMORAL NECK FRACTURES

The aging population faces significant challenges in relation to femoral neck fractures, including:
- *Increased cost of treatment*: There is a high risk of reoperation in the elderly population, leading to overall higher treatment costs.

- *High rate of reoperation*: The reoperation rate for femoral neck fractures can be as high as 34%, adding to the healthcare burden and potentially impacting patient outcomes.
- *Significant loss of function*: Femoral neck fractures can result in decreased mobility, independence in function, and overall quality of life. This may lead to higher rates of institutionalization and the need for assistance with self-care tasks.
- *Impact on health and quality of life*: Patients may experience a decline in function, health, and quality of life following a femoral neck fracture, requiring ongoing care and support.

Addressing these challenges requires effective treatment strategies, such as the use of advanced surgical techniques and implants like the femoral neck system, to improve outcomes and reduce the burden on healthcare systems.

Femoral neck fractures present significant challenges in orthopedic management, accompanied by a spectrum of complications that can impact patient outcomes and prognosis. Understanding these challenges is crucial for guiding treatment decisions and optimizing surgical outcomes.

Avascular necrosis of the femoral head is a serious consequence of NOF fractures. The frequency of AVN varies according to fracture displacement, patient age, and timing of surgery. AVN rates in individuals with misplaced femoral neck fractures have been observed to range between 10 and 30% in studies. Importantly, the timing of surgery plays a critical role in preventing AVN, as early surgical intervention within 24–48 hours has been shown to significantly reduce the risk of AVN development

Additionally, nonunion and malunion are potential complications following femoral neck fractures, particularly in cases of delayed or inadequate treatment. The incidence of nonunion ranges from 5 to 10%, with higher rates observed in displaced fractures and elderly patients. Malunion, less often seen, is characterized by improper alignment or healing of the fractured bone, and can lead to functional impairment and altered biomechanics of the hip joint, predisposing patients to early degenerative changes and osteoarthritis.

Furthermore, postoperative complications such as infection, implant failure, and deep vein thrombosis (DVT) pose significant risks in patients undergoing surgical fixation for femoral neck fractures. The incidence of surgical site infection ranges from 1 to 5%, necessitating prompt diagnosis and appropriate management to prevent further complications. Similarly, DVT and pulmonary embolism (PE) are potential complications associated with prolonged immobilization and surgical trauma, emphasizing the importance of early mobilization and thromboprophylaxis measures.

## Summary

Femoral neck fractures are fraught with challenges and potential complications that necessitate prompt and appropriate management. Early surgical intervention is crucial for reducing the risk of AVN and optimizing outcomes, highlighting the significance of timely evaluation and treatment in this patient population. A comprehensive understanding of the associated complications and their management is essential for trauma surgeons to provide optimal care and improve patient outcomes following femoral neck fractures.

## ■ SUGGESTED READINGS

1. Looker AC, Melton LJ 3rd, Harris TB, Borrud LG, Shepherd JA. Prevalence and trends in low femur bone density among older US adults: NHANES 2005–2006 compared with NHANES III. J Bone Miner Res. 2020;25(1):64-71.
2. Haentjens P, Magaziner J, Colón-Emeric CS, Vanderschueren D, Milisen K, Velkeniers B, et al. Meta-analysis: excess mortality after hip fracture among older women and men. Ann Intern Med. 2010;152(6):380-90.
3. Leal J, Gray AM, Prieto-Alhambra D, Arden NK, Cooper C, Javaid MK, et al.; REFReSH Study Group. Impact of hip fracture on hospital care costs: a population-based study. Osteoporos Int. 2016;27:549-58.
4. George J, Sharma V, Farooque K, Trikha V, Mittal S, Malhotra R. Excess mortality in elderly hip fracture patients: An Indian experience. Chin J Traumatol. 2023;26(6):363-8.
5. Gopalakrishnan A, Sreesobh KV, Jose J. Management of neglected femur neck fractures treated with non vascularised fibular graft. Indian J Orthop Surg. 2018;4(2):160-4.
6. Court-Brown CM, Heckman JD, McQueen MM, Ricci W, Tornetta T, III, McKee MD. Femoral neck fractures. Rockwood and Green's Fractures in Adults, volume 2, 8th edition. Netherlands: Wolters Kluwer; 2015. p. 2037.

# CHAPTER 2

# Anatomy and Biomechanics of the Femoral Neck

*Pramod Bhor, Shivam Mehra, Sushmit Singh, Shikhar D Singh, Sachin Yashwant Kale*

## ■ DETAILED ANATOMY OF THE FEMORAL NECK AND SURROUNDING STRUCTURES

### Introduction

The femoral neck, a crucial anatomical structure linking the femoral head to the femoral shaft, presents challenges in trauma management due to its intricate vascular supply and surrounding ligamentous support. Understanding these anatomical intricacies is paramount for optimal surgical outcomes in femoral neck fractures.

### Blood Supply: MCFA, LCFA and their Importance

The femoral head's blood supply primarily derives from the medial circumflex femoral artery (MCFA), with the lateral circumflex femoral artery (LCFA) providing supplementary support. The MCFA, which originates through the profunda femoris artery, supplies roughly between 70 and 80% of the blood flow to the femoral head, making it susceptible in neck of femur (NOF) fractures. The LCFA, which originates from the femoral artery, acts as an additional source of vascularization, which is especially important in situations with damaged MCFA. Understanding these vascular dynamics is critical because a reduced blood supply raises the likelihood of avascular necrosis (AVN) of the femoral head, necessitating prompt surgery to prevent this problem **(Fig. 1)**.

### Calcar Femorale and its Importance

The calcar femorale, a bony ridge within the femoral neck, plays a vital role in load transmission and fracture stability. Its integrity is crucial in maintaining the mechanical integrity of the femoral neck and preventing displacement of fracture fragments. Preservation of the calcar femorale is thus a key consideration in surgical management, as its disruption may lead to increased risk of nonunion and malunion in femoral neck fractures.

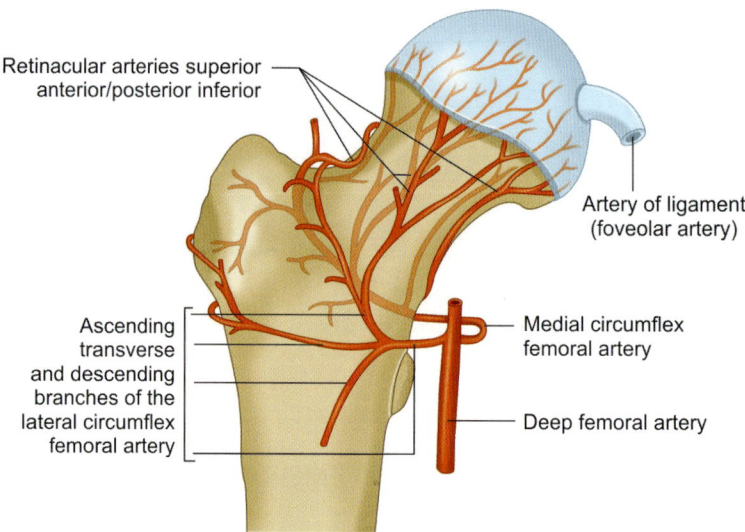

**FIG. 1:** Blood supply of proximal femur.
*Source*: Lu Y, Uppal HS. Hip fractures: relevant anatomy, classification, and biomechanics of fracture and fixation. Geriatric orthopedic surgery and rehabilitation. 2019;10:2151459319859139.

### Capsule of Hip Joint and its Importance

The femoral capsule, a dense fibrous structure enveloping the hip joint, contributes significantly to its stability. Disruption of the capsule in femoral neck fractures can lead to joint instability and compromise fracture healing. Additionally, the capsule's integrity influences the timing of surgery, as early intervention is essential to restore joint stability and minimize the risk of nonunion. Understanding the role of the hip capsule is crucial in surgical decision-making, emphasizing the importance of timely intervention to optimize patient outcomes.

### Summary

An understanding of the femoral neck's intricate vascular supply, bony architecture, and surrounding soft tissues is crucial for trauma surgeons managing femoral neck fractures. Appreciating the significance of these anatomical structures guides surgical decision-making, minimizing complications such as AVN and nonunion, and optimizing patient outcomes.

## ■ BIOMECHANICAL PRINCIPLES RELEVANT TO FEMORAL NECK FRACTURES AND FIXATION

Biomechanical principles are pivotal in understanding the behavior of femoral neck fractures and guiding optimal fixation strategies. The femoral neck experiences complex loading patterns, necessitating consideration of biomechanical factors in fracture management.

The Pauwels' classification method classifies NOF fractures according to the inclination of the fracture line compared to the plane of horizontal extension. Fractures with larger shear angles, known as Pauwels type III, have been linked with increased instabilities and fixation failure. Studies have shown failure rates of up to 40% in fractures with high shear angles, emphasizing the importance of selecting appropriate fixation methods based on fracture morphology.

Following femoral neck fractures, muscle forces can contribute to deformities such as varus or valgus angulation. The hip abductor muscles, including the gluteus medius and minimus, may cause varus deformity by pulling the femoral shaft superiorly, while the hip adductor muscles, including the adductor magnus and longus, may produce valgus deformity by exerting a medial force on the femoral shaft. Understanding the biomechanics of muscle action is essential for predicting and managing postfracture deformities.

Various fixation methods, including dynamic hip screws, cannulated screws, and sliding hip screws, exhibit distinct biomechanical strengths. Dynamic hip screws provide stable fixation by resisting shear and rotational forces, with biomechanical studies demonstrating superior resistance to varus collapse compared to other fixation methods. Cannulated screws offer reliable fixation by compressing fracture fragments, while sliding hip screws provide excellent resistance to axial and rotational forces. Biomechanical studies comparing fixation methods have shown varying degrees of stability and resistance to failure, highlighting the importance of selecting the most appropriate technique based on fracture characteristics and patient factors.

## Summary

Biomechanical principles inform the selection of fixation methods and guide surgical decision-making in femoral neck fractures. By considering factors such as fracture morphology, muscle forces, and implant biomechanics, surgeons can optimize treatment strategies to achieve stable fixation and promote successful fracture healing.

## ■ UNDERSTANDING LOAD-BEARING CAPACITY AND STRESS DISTRIBUTION IN THE FEMORAL NECK

The femoral neck's load-bearing capacity is a critical aspect of its biomechanical function. Studies have shown that the femoral neck can withstand compressive loads of up to 2,000–2,500 N and tensile loads of approximately 1,000 N before failure occurs. This highlights the femoral neck's ability to withstand substantial forces during weight-bearing activities.

Primary tensile and compressive lines in the femoral neck and intertrochanteric region influence stress distribution. The femoral neck is subjected to primary compressive forces along its inferomedial aspect and primary tensile forces along its superolateral aspect. Similarly, the intertrochanteric region experiences primary compressive forces along the calcar femorale and primary tensile forces along the intertrochanteric line. Understanding these force vectors is crucial for comprehending fracture patterns and guiding surgical fixation techniques.

The posterior medial part of the femoral neck is anatomically the strongest region, characterized by dense cortical bone and optimal trabecular architecture. Consequently, implants placed in this region, such as dynamic hip screws or cannulated screws, benefit from the best cortical purchase, enhancing stability and reducing the risk of implant failure. This strategic placement exploits the femoral neck's inherent biomechanical properties to maximize fixation strength.

The neck-shaft angle, typically ranging from 120° to 140°, plays a crucial role in load distribution and biomechanical stability. A decreased neck-shaft angle, termed coxa vara, shifts the center of gravity laterally, increasing the mechanical stress on the femoral neck and predisposing individuals to fracture. Conversely, an increased neck-shaft angle, termed coxa valga, may alter force transmission, affecting joint biomechanics and increasing the risk of femoral neck fractures. Therefore, accurate assessment of the neck-shaft angle is essential for evaluating fracture stability and guiding surgical management decisions.

## Summary

Understanding the load-bearing capacity, stress distribution, and anatomical characteristics of the femoral neck is crucial for effective management of femoral neck fractures. By considering factors such as force vectors, bone strength, and anatomical variations, clinicians can optimize surgical techniques and implant placement to achieve optimal outcomes and reduce the risk of complications.

## ■ SUGGESTED READINGS

1. Gurusamy K, Parker MJ, Rowlands TK. The complications of displaced intracapsular fractures of the hip: the effect of screw positioning and angulation on fracture healing. J Bone Joint Surg. 2005;87(5):632-4.
2. Konda SR, Johnson JR, Kelly EA, Chan J, Lyon T, Egol KA. Can we accurately predict which geriatric and middle-aged hip fracture patients will experience a delay to surgery? Geriatr Orthop Surg Rehabil. 2020;11:2151459320946021.
3. Giannoudis PV, Kontakis G, Christoforakis Z, Akula M, Tosounidis T, Koutras C. Management, complications and clinical results of femoral head fractures. Injury. 2009;40(12):1245-51.
4. Stoffel K, Zderic I, Gras F, Sommer C, Eberli U, Mueller D, et al. Biomechanical Evaluation of the Femoral Neck System in Unstable Pauwels III Femoral Neck Fractures: A Comparison with the Dynamic Hip Screw and Cannulated Screws. J Orthop Trauma. 2017;31(3):131-7.

# CHAPTER 3

# Evolution of Femoral Neck System Implants

*Sanjay Dhar, Gaurav Kanade, Arvind J Vatkar, Sachin Yashwant Kale*

## ■ HISTORICAL OVERVIEW OF FEMORAL NECK FRACTURE TREATMENT METHODS

Femoral neck fracture treatment has evolved significantly over time. Initially managed conservatively with bed rest and traction, historical methods yielded high rates of complications. Conservative approaches led to up to 30% nonunion as well as 20–30% avascular necrosis (AVN).

The evolution of neck femur fixation implants, particularly for fractures of the femoral neck, reflects significant advancements in materials, design, and surgical techniques. Over the years the key developments that have occurred have moved from simple mechanical devices to sophisticated systems designed to optimize stability, promote healing, and minimize complications.

### Early Fixation Techniques

*Traction and casting*: Before the development of internal fixation methods, femoral neck fractures were treated nonsurgically with traction and casting, often leading to poor outcomes due to prolonged immobilization and limited ability to achieve stable fixation.

*Introduction of internal fixation*: The late 19th century saw the introduction of surgical procedures such as open reduction and internal fixation, also known as ORIF, with metal pins, wires, and plates. Subsequent developments included dynamic hip screws (DHS) and cannulated screws, which reduced nonunion rates to 5–10% and AVN rates to 10–20%.

*Screws and pins (1930s–1940s)*: Early internal fixation methods included the use of simple screws and pins. The Smith–Petersen nail, introduced in the 1930s, was one of the first intramedullary devices designed to provide internal support for hip fractures.

*Garden screw*: Developed by RS Garden in the 1950s, this large cancellous screw was specifically designed for femoral neck fractures, allowing for compression at the fracture site and improved stability **(Fig. 1)**.

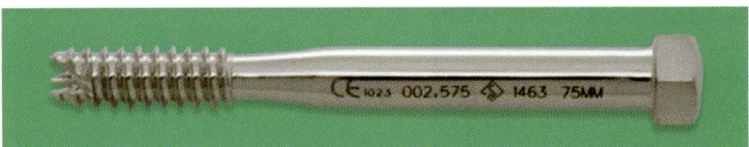

**FIG. 1:** Garden screw.

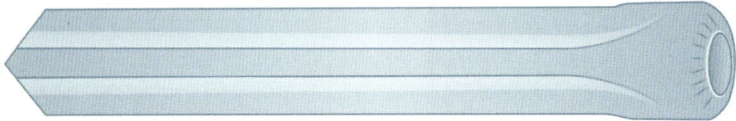

**FIG. 2:** Smith–Peterson nail.

In the 1950s the sliding hip screw (SHS) was developed. The term SHS is synonymous with the term compression hip screw and equivalent models, such as the Dynamic, Richards and Ambi hip screws. These are considered "dynamic" implants as they have the capacity for sliding at the plate/screw junction to allow for collapse at the fracture site. Early implants were based on a Smith–Peterson nail to which was attached a side plate. These implants **(Fig. 2)** are termed "static" or "fixed" implants (FNP) as they have no capacity for sliding.

*Dynamic hip screw (1960s)*: The introduction of the DHS revolutionized the treatment of femoral neck fractures. It consists of a large screw that slides within a barrel attached to a side plate, allowing for controlled compression at the fracture site during weight-bearing. This system offered improved stability and promoted early mobilization of patients.

### Cannulated Screw Systems

*Cannulated screws (1980s-1990s)*: These screws, which have a hollow core, allow for more precise placement using guide wires. Multiple cannulated screws can be placed in various configurations to achieve stable fixation while preserving bone stock.

*Femoral neck system* (FNS) is a modified sliding screw allowing better controlled fixation and sliding to provide controlled compression at the fracture site.

The FNS, which is a minimally invasive implant recently developed for the treatment of femoral neck fractures, including basilar, transcervical, and subcapital fractures, combines the advantages of angular stability with the minimally invasive surgical technique.

Various studies have shown FNS biomechanical stability comparable to the DHS and superior to cannulated screws in unstable Pauwels III femoral neck fractures in normal bone; however, in *osteoporotic bones* studies have yet to prove it.

The ease of placing a single guide wire in the neck and allowing the derotation screw provides some technical advantages over the DHS.

Modern implants FNS offer improved biomechanical stability and facilitate earlier mobilization, leading to better outcomes and reduced complications compared to conservative management.

## ■ INTRODUCTION TO THE CONCEPT OF MODERN IMPLANTS AND THEIR EVOLUTION

The evolution of implants for femoral neck fractures has significantly advanced fracture management. In the late 19th century, early implants such as pins, wires, and plates were introduced, providing stabilization but often leading to complications like implant failure and infection.

In the mid-20th century, DHS emerged as a popular choice, offering improved biomechanical stability and reduced rates of nonunion. However, drawbacks included limited rotational stability and risk of implant cut-out in unstable fractures.

Cannulated screws have also been widely used, offering precise implant placement and good fixation. However, they may not provide adequate rotational stability in certain fracture patterns.

Recently, the FNS implant has been developed, combining the benefits of multiple fixation methods. FNS implants offer improved biomechanical properties, rotational stability, and versatility in fracture management, representing a promising advancement in femoral neck fracture treatment.

## ■ COMPARATIVE ANALYSIS OF VARIOUS FIXATION METHODS AND THEIR OUTCOMES

Comparing fixation methods for femoral neck fractures provides insights into their efficacy and outcomes. DHS with derotation screws offer good biomechanical stability, reducing nonunion rates to approximately 5–10% and malunion rates to 5–15%. However, rotational stability remains a concern.

Cannulated compression screws (CCS) provide precise fixation and improved rotational stability but may not offer adequate biomechanical strength in unstable fractures. Complication rates range from 10 to 20%, with risks of implant cut-out and nonunion.

The FNS implant, a recent innovation, combines the advantages of multiple fixation methods, offering enhanced biomechanical stability and versatility. Comparative studies have shown reduced complication rates compared to traditional methods, with nonunion rates ranging from 2 to 5%.

Biomechanically, FNS implants demonstrate superior rotational stability and load-bearing capacity compared to DHS and CCS screws. However, long-term outcomes and complication rates require further investigation to establish the superiority of FNS implants in femoral neck fracture management.

## Summary

Treatment methods for femoral neck fractures have evolved from conservative approaches to advanced surgical techniques. Initially managed with bed rest and traction, early methods led to high rates of nonunion (up to 30%) and avascular necrosis (20–30%). The late 19th century introduced internal fixation with metal pins, wires, and plates, improving outcomes. In the mid-20th century, dynamic hip screws (DHS) and cannulated screws were developed, further reducing complications. The DHS, introduced in the 1960s, provided controlled compression and stability, promoting early mobilization. In the 1980s–1990s, cannulated screws allowed precise placement, preserving bone stock. The recent femoral neck system (FNS) combines advantages of multiple fixation methods, offering enhanced biomechanical stability and versatility. Studies suggest FNS implants reduce complication rates and provide better outcomes, though long-term data is still needed.

## ■ SUGGESTED READINGS

1. Tidermark J, Ponzer S, Svensson O, Söderqvist A, Törnkvist H. Internal fixation compared with total hip replacement for displaced femoral neck fractures in the elderly: A randomised, controlled trial. J Bone Joint Surg. 2003;85(3):380-8.
2. Schipper IB, Steyerberg EW, Castelein RM, Van der Heijden FH, Den Hoed PT, Kerver AJ, et al. Treatment of unstable trochanteric fractures: Randomised comparison of the gamma nail and the proximal femoral nail. J Bone Joint Surg. 2004;86(1):86-94.
3. Parker MJ, Gurusamy KS, Azegami S. Arthroplasties (with and without bone cement) for proximal femoral fractures in adults. Cochrane Database Syst Rev. 2010(6):CD001706.
4. Bretherton CP, Parker MJ. Femoral medialization, fixation failures, and functional outcome in trochanteric hip fractures treated with either a sliding hip screw or an intramedullary nail from within a randomized trial. J Orthop Trauma. 2016;30(12):642-6.
5. Stoffel K, Zderic I, Gras F, Sommer C, Eberli U, Mueller D, et al. Biomechanical Evaluation of the Femoral Neck System in Unstable Pauwels III Femoral Neck Fractures: A Comparison with the Dynamic Hip Screw and Cannulated Screws. J Orthop Trauma. 2017;31(3):131-7.

# CHAPTER 4

# Design Principles and Components of Femoral Neck System Implants

Ansh Gupta, Sandeep Patel, Ajit Chalak, Arvind J Vatkar, Sunil Shetty, Vishal Kumar

## ■ A SUMMARY OF THE DESIGN CHARACTERISTICS OF FEMORAL NECK SYSTEM IMPLANTS

The femoral neck system (FNS), developed by DePuy Synthes, represents a significant advancement in the surgical management of femoral neck fractures. Designed with innovative features, the FNS prioritizes biomechanical stability, versatility, and ease of implantation.

The system comprises three components: A base plate, a femoral neck bolt, and an antirotation screw. The two-holed base plate offers a small implant footprint in comparison to the conventional sliding hip screw barrel plates. It also facilitates the insertion of the antirotation screw through the same hole, avoiding the need for further dissection proximally. The small low-profile plate reduces lateral protrusion, bursitis, and lateral hip pain. The femoral neck bolt is the main working component of the FNS system. It acts as the central load carrier and offloads the fracture. The 10 mm bolt has a neck shaft angle of 130° to the base plate; however, it allows a placement of ± 5°. The bolt glides freely in the barrel enabling a controlled collapse of 20 mm. It has a blunt tip unlike the conventional cannulated screws, decreasing the chance of an articular cut-out. Similar to the sliding hip screw, it ought to be put in the middle of the femoral neck, somewhat inferior to the apex of the femoral head. The antirotation screw is 6.4 mm in diameter and forks out at a 5° angle from the bolt's base. Its divergence from the bolt generates rotational resistance.

The screw is locked with the neck bolt making the whole structure one single construct capable of sliding in the barrel leading. This makes it a dynamic fixed angle construct. The minimum size of the bolt screw system is 75 mm and is available in 5 mm increments. However, if the anatomy demands a shorter screw, a 70 mm construct can be made with 15 mm sliding potential **(Fig. 1)**.

# CHAPTER 4: Design Principles and Components of Femoral Neck System Implants

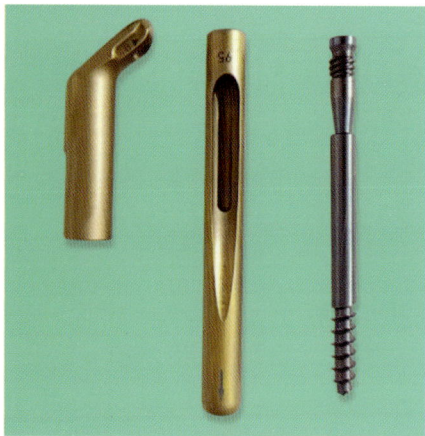

**FIG. 1:** The femoral neck system.

The FNS system, similar to the sliding hip screw, works on the principle of controlled collapse. It allows dynamic compression of the neck while simultaneously preventing collapse upon varus with weight-bearing. It has quicker time to union, less incidence of femoral shortening, and better functional outcomes.

One of the key design principles of the FNS is its modularity, allowing for customization to accommodate various fracture patterns and patient anatomy. The system comprises interchangeable components, including screws, plates, and locking mechanisms, enabling surgeons to tailor fixation based on individual patient factors.

The FNS offers several advantages over traditional fixation methods such as dynamic hip screws (DHS) and cannulated compression screws (CCS). Its locking mechanism provides enhanced rotational stability, reducing the risk of implant failure and malunion. Additionally, the FNS facilitates minimally invasive surgery with smaller incisions and reduced soft-tissue disruption, leading to faster recovery times and improved patient outcomes compared to DHS and CCS.

Furthermore, the FNS's streamlined instrumentation simplifies surgical procedures, allowing for efficient implantation and reduced operative times. Its anatomically contoured plates and screws optimize bone purchase and fixation strength, minimizing the risk of complications such as implant cut-out and nonunion **(Fig. 2)**.

## Summary

The FNS's design features, including modularity, locking mechanism, and minimally invasive approach, offer distinct advantages over traditional fixation methods. By prioritizing biomechanical stability and surgical efficiency, the FNS represents a significant advancement in femoral neck fracture management, improving outcomes and patient satisfaction.

# CHAPTER 4: Design Principles and Components of Femoral Neck System Implants

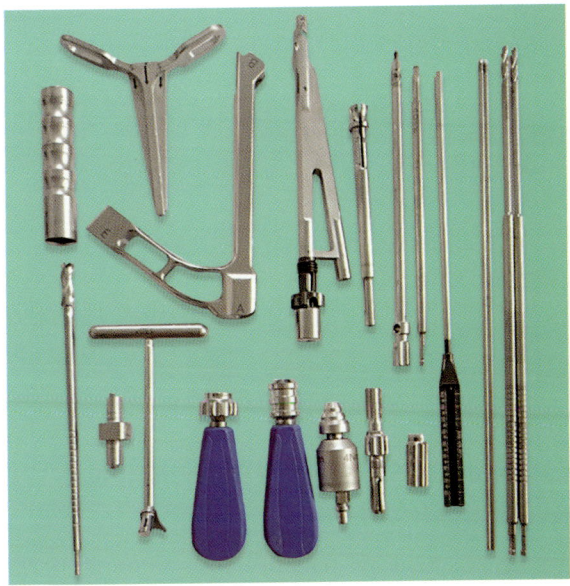

**FIG. 2:** Instrumentation set for femoral neck system.

## ■ SUGGESTED READINGS

1. Stoffel K, Sommer C. Femoral Neck System. [online] Available from https://www.aofoundation.org/approved/approvedsolutionsfolder/2017/femoral-neck-system#tab=details [Last accessed July, 2024].
2. Stoffel K, Zderic I, Gras F, Sommer C, Eberli U, Mueller D, et al. Biomechanical Evaluation of the Femoral Neck System in Unstable Pauwels III Femoral Neck Fractures: A Comparison with the Dynamic Hip Screw and Cannulated Screws. J Orthop Trauma. 2017;31(3):131-7.
3. Lu Y, Canavese F, Nan G, Lin R, Huang Y, Pan N, et al. Is Femoral Neck System a Valid Alternative for the Treatment of Displaced Femoral Neck Fractures in Adolescents? A Comparative Study of Femoral Neck System versus Cannulated Compression Screw. Medicina (Kaunas). 2022;58(8):999.
4. Patel S, Kumar V, Baburaj V, Dhillon MS. The use of the femoral neck system (FNS) leads to better outcomes in the surgical management of femoral neck fractures in adults compared to fixation with cannulated screws: A systematic review and meta-analysis. Eur J Orthop Surg Traumatol. 2023;33(5):2101-9.

# CHAPTER 5

# Preoperative Evaluation and Surgical Planning

*Gaurav Kanade, Sachin Yashwant Kale, Sanjay Dhar, Aditya R Gunjotikar*

## ■ COMPREHENSIVE ASSESSMENT OF PATIENTS WITH FEMORAL NECK FRACTURES

Comprehensive assessment of patients with femoral neck fractures is essential for guiding treatment decisions and optimizing outcomes, following protocols similar to those outlined in the Advanced Trauma Life Support (ATLS) guidelines. This assessment encompasses various aspects, including patient history, physical examination, imaging studies, and consideration of comorbidities.

Patients' medical history should include evaluation for osteoporosis, as it significantly influences fracture risk and management strategies. Identification of preexisting conditions such as diabetes, cardiovascular disease, and neurological disorders is crucial for assessing perioperative risks and planning appropriate care.

Radiographic evaluation is vital for determining fracture patterns, including subcapital, transcervical, and basicervical fractures, as well as associated injuries such as acetabular or pelvic fractures. Moreover, measuring the angle of the femoral neck fracture, such as the neck-shaft angle, aids in predicting stability and guiding surgical decision-making.

In addition to assessing the femoral neck fracture itself, evaluation for other concurrent fractures, particularly in the pelvis and lower extremities, is essential for comprehensive management. Recognition of associated injuries impacts treatment plans, rehabilitation strategies, and overall prognosis.

Overall, a thorough and systematic assessment of patients with femoral neck fractures, considering osteoporosis, preexisting diseases, fracture patterns, and associated injuries is crucial for delivering optimal care and achieving favorable outcomes. This multidimensional approach ensures tailored management strategies that address individual patient needs and mitigate potential complications.

A complete evaluation of patients with neck of femur (NOF) fractures is required for efficient therapy using the femoral neck system (FNS).

A complete health history, physical examination, and diagnostic imaging tests should be performed to evaluate the nature of the fracture as well as any accompanying injuries or medical disorders. When establishing the best treatment approach, it is also important to consider the patient's aging, functional level, and bone condition. Imaging tests such as X-rays, computed tomography (CT) scans, and magnetic resonance imaging (MRI) can offer extensive information regarding fracture pattern, displacement, and bone health.

Additionally, laboratory tests like blood work and urinalysis can help identify any underlying medical conditions that may affect treatment outcomes. The assessment should also include a functional evaluation to determine the patient's ability to perform daily activities and assess the potential impact of the fracture on their quality of life. By conducting a comprehensive assessment, surgeons can develop a personalized treatment plan that addresses the patient's unique needs and optimizes outcomes using the FNS.

## Summary

Comprehensive assessment of patients with femoral neck fractures is crucial for optimal treatment and outcomes, following protocols similar to Advanced Trauma Life Support (ATLS) guidelines. This involves a thorough medical history, physical examination, and imaging studies, considering factors like osteoporosis and comorbidities. Radiographic evaluation determines fracture patterns and stability, while also identifying concurrent injuries. A multidimensional approach, including functional and laboratory assessments, tailors management strategies to individual patient needs, ensuring effective therapy and minimizing complications.

## ■ RADIOLOGICAL EVALUATION TECHNIQUES AND THEIR ROLE IN SURGICAL PLANNING

Radiological evaluation plays a pivotal role in surgical planning for femoral neck fractures, aiding in fracture classification, assessment of displacement, and evaluation of associated injuries. X-rays are the initial imaging modality of choice, providing valuable information about fracture patterns, displacement, and alignment. Traction X-ray views of hips can also help to see fracture patterns. They allow for the determination of critical factors such as the angle of the fracture of the neck of the femur and the degree of comminution at the fracture site, which influence treatment decisions.

Computed tomography scans offer enhanced visualization of fracture anatomy and are particularly useful for assessing complex fractures, including those with intra-articular extension or significant comminution. CT imaging provides detailed information about fracture patterns, intra-articular involvement, and degree of osteoporosis, facilitating precise surgical planning and implant selection.

Moreover, CT scans aid in evaluating the integrity of the surrounding bone and soft tissues, identifying associated injuries such as pelvic fractures or acetabular involvement. This comprehensive assessment guides the surgeons in determining the most appropriate surgical approach, fixation technique, and implant selection to optimize fracture reduction and stability.

## Summary

Radiological evaluation techniques, including X-rays and CT scans, are indispensable tools in surgical planning for femoral neck fractures. They provide crucial information about fracture morphology, displacement, osteoporosis, and associated injuries, enabling surgeons to make informed decisions and achieve optimal outcomes for patients undergoing surgical intervention.

## ■ CONSIDERATIONS FOR PATIENT-SPECIFIC FACTORS AND SURGICAL APPROACH SELECTION

Tailoring the management of femoral neck fractures to patient-specific factors is crucial for optimizing surgical outcomes. Age, functional status, comorbidities, fracture characteristics, and osteoporosis all play vital roles in treatment decisions and surgical approach selection.

Elderly patients, particularly those with low functional demands and significant medical comorbidities, may benefit from hemiarthroplasty to facilitate early mobilization and reduce perioperative morbidity. This approach offers reliable pain relief and allows for swift rehabilitation, promoting better overall outcomes in this population.

Fracture displacement, angulation, and comminution also influence surgical decision-making. Displaced fractures with significant displacement or intra-articular involvement may necessitate open reduction techniques to achieve anatomical reduction and stability. Conversely, minimally displaced fractures or those with minimal comminution may be amenable to percutaneous or closed reduction methods.

Moreover, considering the impact of preexisting osteoporosis on implant selection and fixation stability is crucial. Patients with severe osteoporosis may require augmented fixation techniques, such as cement augmentation or the use of implants specifically designed for osteoporotic bone.

## Summary

Individualized treatment strategies based on patient-specific factors, fracture characteristics, and bone quality are essential for optimizing outcomes in femoral neck fractures. Tailoring the surgical approach to each patient's needs ensures the best possible functional recovery and long-term success, particularly in the elderly population requiring early mobilization.

# CHAPTER 5: Preoperative Evaluation and Surgical Planning

## ■ SUGGESTED READING

1. Pauyo T, Drager J, Albers A, Harvey EJ. Management of femoral neck fractures in the young patient. Clin Orthop Relat Res. 2014;472(6):1941-52.
2. Parker MJ, Gurusamy KS. Internal fixation versus arthroplasty for intracapsular proximal femoral fractures in adults. Cochrane Database Syst Rev. 2006;2006(4): CD001708.
3. Lawrence JE, Fountain DM, Cundall-Curry DJ, Carrothers AD. Do patients with hip fractures benefit from orthogeriatric care? An observational study of 13,731 patients in a UK hip fracture unit. Injury. 2017;48(7):1468-74.
4. Bhandari M, Devereaux PJ, Tornetta P, Swiontkowski MF, Berry DJ, Haidukewych G, et al. Operative management of displaced femoral neck fractures in elderly patients: An international survey. J Bone Joint Surg Am. 2005;87(9):2122-30.
5. Kain MS, Marcantonio AJ, Iorio R. Surgical management of hip fractures: An evidence-based review of the literature. II: Intertrochanteric fractures. J Am Acad Orthop Surg. 2014;22(11):665-73.

# CHAPTER 6

# Step-by-Step Guide to Surgical Procedures for Femoral Neck Fracture Fixation

Sachin Yashwant Kale, Prasad Liladhar Chaudhari, Arvind J Vatkar, Shikhar D Singh

## ■ SURGICAL APPROACHES, POSITIONING, AND INTRAOPERATIVE CONSIDERATIONS

Patients undergoing this procedure are administered suitable anesthesia and positioned in supine position on an Orthopedic traction table.

The fractured neck is meticulously realigned to restore its optimal anatomical orientation, employing the capabilities of the traction table.

If there is inability to achieve a closed reduction, open reduction is mandatory (Watson–Jones approach) as an anatomical reduction is a prerequisite for starting the procedure.

To maintain the highest standards of asepsis, the surgical field is prepared, involving the application of antiseptic solutions, scrubbing, and placement of sterile drapes.

To aid in reducing and stabilizing of the fracture, mild traction is used, which entails gradual movements in flexion, adduction, abduction, and internal rotation of roughly 15 degrees, while maintaining the neck of the femur parallel to the operating table

Reduction confirm in both AP and LAT views under C Arm **(Figs. 1A and B)**.

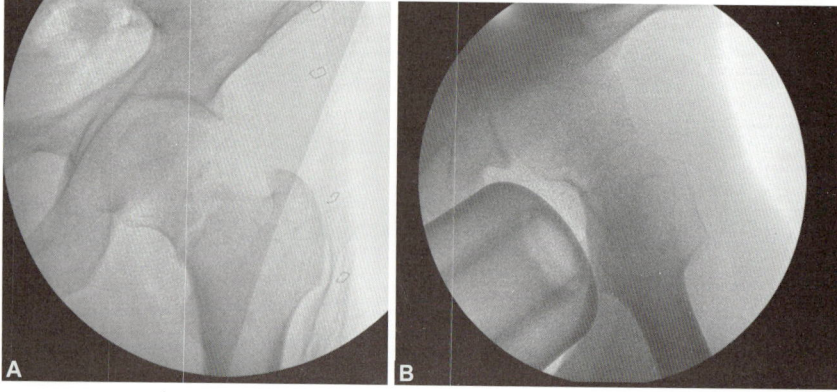

**FIGS. 1A AND B:** Reduction confirm in both anterior-posterior (AP) and lateral (LAT) views.

# CHAPTER 6: Step-by-Step Guide to Surgical Procedures for Femoral Neck...

A transverse incision of about 4–5 cm is carefully made below the greater trochanter, along the shaft of femoral bone **(Fig. 2)**.

A 4–5 cm transverse incision is made from the greater trochanter along the shaft of the femur. Incision deepened to exposed the tensor fascia lata. TFL incised to expose the bone. A guidewire placed in the centre of the femoral head in both AP and lateral views with the help of an angle guide **(Figs. 3A to D)**.

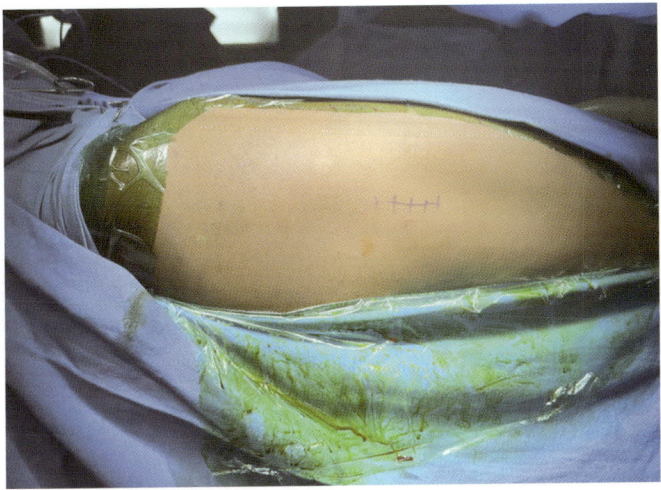

**FIG. 2:** A transverse incision of about 4 cm is carefully made below the greater trochanter, allowing entry to the lateral compartments of the femoral bone.

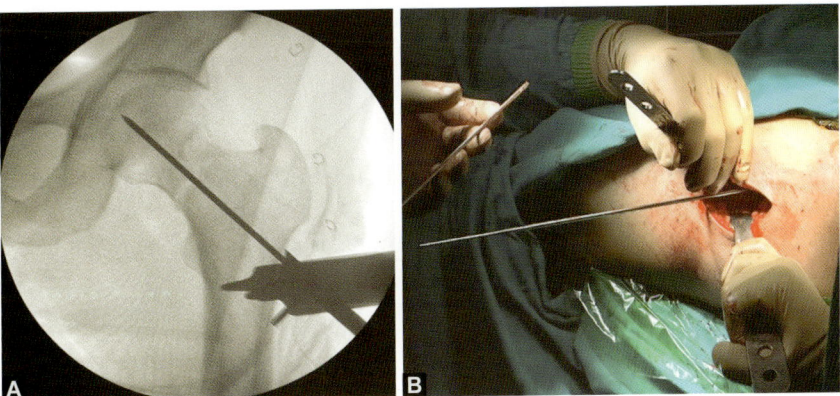

**FIGS. 3A TO D:** *Continued*

*Continued*

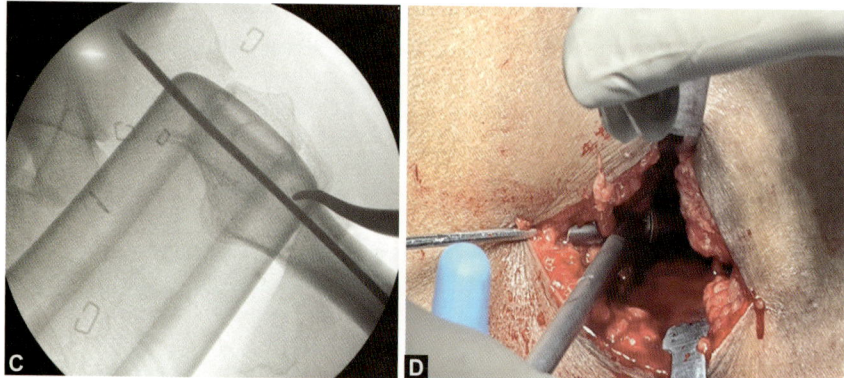

**FIGS. 3A TO D:** Guidewire placed in the center of the head; anterior-posterior (AP) and lateral views and clinical picture.

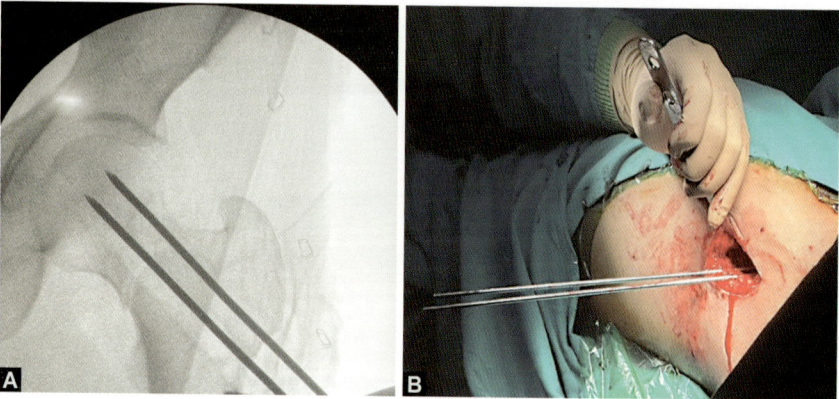

**FIGS. 4A AND B:** To prevent the femoral head from rotating unintentionally, a derotation guidewire is placed either via a lateral incision or percutaneously into the superior and anterior regions of the femoral neck.

To prevent the femoral head from rotating unintentionally, a derotation guide wire is placed either via a lateral incision or percutaneously into the superior and anterior region of the femoral neck under C-arm guidance **(Figs. 4A and B)**.

Reaming done under C-arm guidance to ensure there is no displacement at the fracture site **(Figs. 5A to C)**.

Precise measurements are taken to determine the required length and select the appropriate femoral neck system implant, aided by a direct measuring instrument. The implant is then carefully introduced into the pre-reamed hole over the central guidewire **(Figs. 6A and B)**.

# CHAPTER 6: Step-by-Step Guide to Surgical Procedures for Femoral Neck...

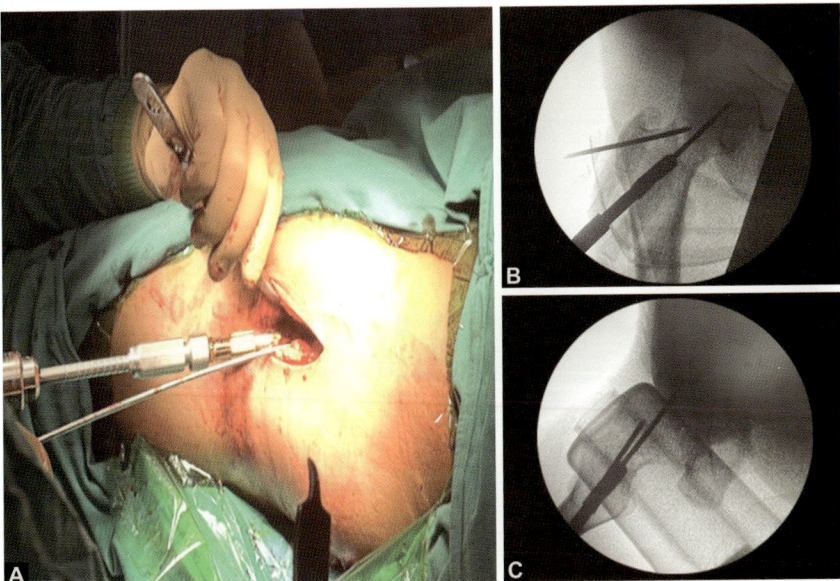

**FIGS. 5A TO C:** Reaming done.

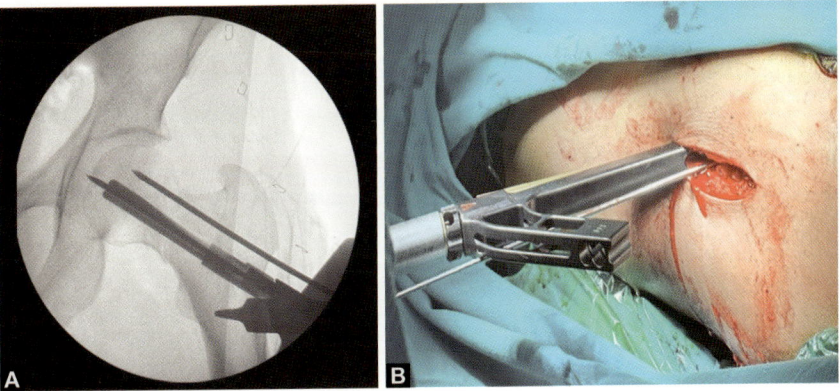

**FIGS. 6A AND B:** Precise measurements are taken to determine the required length and select the appropriate femoral neck system, aided by a direct measuring instrument. The implant is then carefully introduced into the pre-reamed hole over the central guidewire.

Top screw inserted and shaft screw drilling done and after proper measurement shaft screw pass **(Figs. 7A to C)**.

Shaft screw placed and derotation screw passed to complete the procedure **(Figs. 8A and B)**.

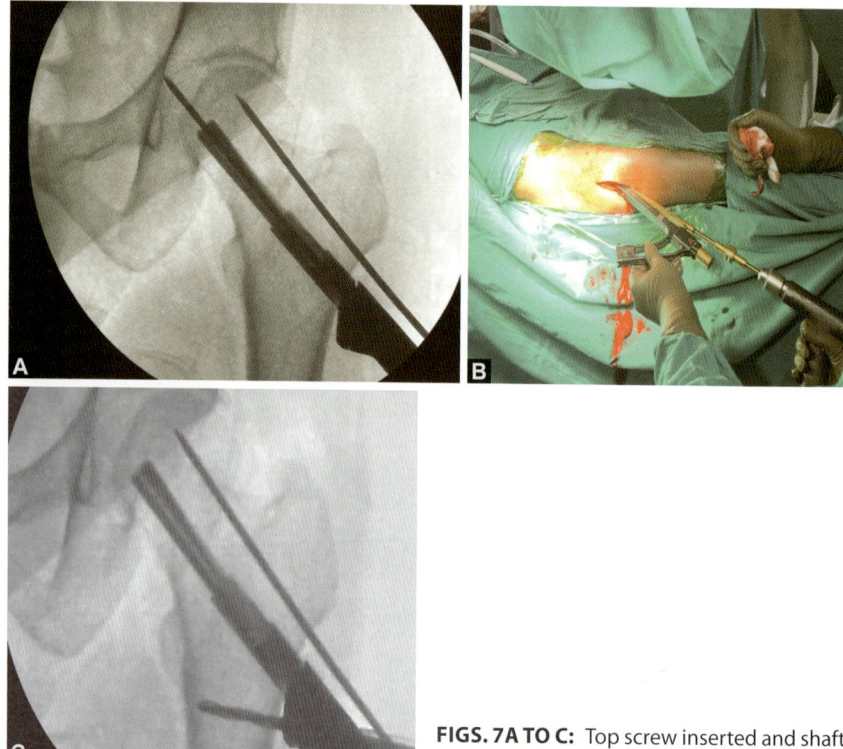

**FIGS. 7A TO C:** Top screw inserted and shaft screw drilling done.

**FIGS. 8A AND B:** Shaft screw placed and derotation screw passed to complete the procedure.

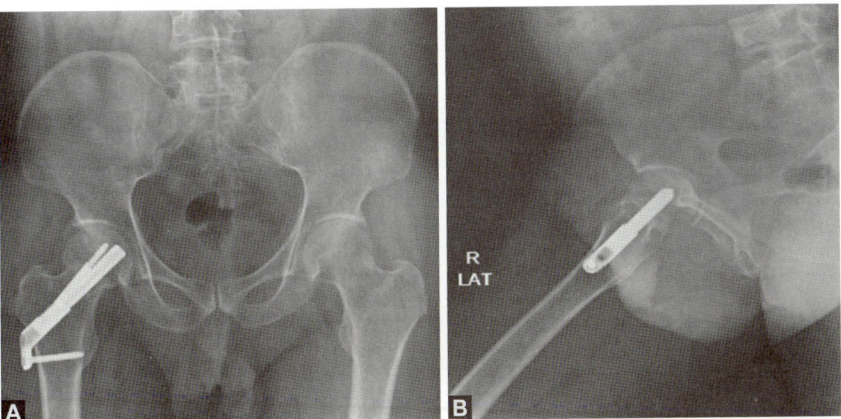

**FIGS. 9A AND B:** Postoperative X-rays.

Final post operative X-rays showing good reduction and proper placement of implant **(Figs. 9A and B)**.

## Summary

The step-by-step guide to femoral neck fracture fixation involves positioning the patient supine on a fracture table with spinal anesthesia. If closed reduction is unsuccessful, an open reduction via the Watson–Jones approach is performed. A 4 cm transverse incision below the greater trochanter allows access for guidewire placement and reaming. The fracture is realigned and the appropriate implant is introduced. Precise measurements ensure proper implant selection, with subsequent insertion of the top screw, shaft screw, and derotation screw, followed by postoperative X-rays to confirm reduction.

### ■ SUGGESTED READINGS

1. Zhang C. Hip Surgery: A Practical Guide. Singapore: Springer Nature; 2020.
2. Kale S, Mishra R, Singh S, Chalak A, Vatkar A, Ghodke R, et al. A prospective study to analyze the functional outcome of the femoral neck system in femoral neck fractures. MGM J Med Sci. 2023;10(3):409-14.

# CHAPTER 7

# Postoperative Care and Rehabilitation Protocols

Shivam Mehra, Nindiya Kapoor Mehra, Pramod Bhor, Aditya R Gunjotikar

## ■ IMMEDIATE POSTOPERATIVE MANAGEMENT STRATEGIES

### Phase 1: Immediate Postoperative Care (Days 1–7)

In the initial postoperative phase, patients are closely observed to manage pain effectively and initiate early mobilization.

*Pain management*: Administer analgesics judiciously to ensure the patient's comfort.

*Reducing joint rigidity and enhanced blood circulation*: These encompass ankle pumps, delicate hip flexion, abduction, and rotation.

*Respiratory health*: Promote deep inhalation and productive coughing routines to avoid respiratory complications.

## ■ REHABILITATION GUIDELINES FOR EARLY MOBILIZATION AND FUNCTIONAL RECOVERY

### Phase 2: Early Mobilization (Days 7–14)

*Weight-bearing progression*: Weight-bearing allowances are individualized based on the fixation, but nil weight-bearing walk is more or less started by postoperative day 7 depending on the patient's pain tolerance. Partial weight-bearing may be allowed with the aid of assistive devices, contingent upon the surgical intervention and implant configuration.

*Range of motion exercises*: Subjects are recommended to participate in a gentle passive range of motion activities. The gradual easing of weight-bearing limitations may be commenced.

*Ambulation training*: Initiate gait rehabilitation under the guidance of a physical therapist. The patient may begin using a walker or crutches with limited load-bearing.

*Strength training*: Inaugurate gentle isometric exercises and low resistance muscle strengthening routines for the hip and lower limb musculature.

## Phase 3: Intermediate Phase (Weeks 2–6)

*Full weight-bearing*: Transition to full weight-bearing in accordance with the surgeon's recommendation. Continued vigilance for correct gait patterns and posture is paramount.

*Progressive strengthening*: Continue progressive resistance regimens to enhance muscle robustness and joint steadiness. Emphasis should be placed on the development of hip abductors, adductors, flexors, and extensors.

*Balance and coordination*: Integrate balance and coordination exercises to refine proprioception and diminish the risk of accidental falls.

*Functional activities*: Encourage patients to practice activities of daily living, including sitting, standing and chair climbing.

## Phase 4: Advanced Rehabilitation (Weeks 6 and Beyond)

*Advanced strengthening*: Escalate resistance and intensity during strengthening exercises.

## ■ MONITORING FOR COMPLICATIONS AND LONG-TERM FOLLOW-UP RECOMMENDATIONS

Chronic obstructive pulmonary disease (COPD), Alzheimer's disease, heart failure, and cancer have all been linked to higher death rates in the months following hip fracture surgery. Prolonged hypoxemia and long-term use of steroids can lead to delayed fracture and healing of wounds. Handling such comorbidities and following up is critical.

Following discharge, the key objective is to manage comorbidities, multiple medications, coordination and equilibrium training, and the patient's surroundings. However, following up on pathological fractures is critical for detecting and treating the root causes, as well as preventing future fractures. Surgeons also play a crucial role in ensuring proper contact with other specialties (such as oncology, hematology, and cardiology), supporting in the coordination of social and community care, and providing advice on mobilization.

## Summary

Immediate postoperative management for femoral neck fractures focuses on pain control, early mobilization, and respiratory health. In the first week, pain is managed with analgesics, and exercises like ankle pumps and gentle hip movements are introduced. From days 7–14, patients begin weight-bearing with assistive devices and engage in range of motion and strength training exercises. Weeks 2–6 involve transitioning to full weight-bearing, progressive strengthening, and balance exercises. Advanced rehabilitation from week 6 onwards includes increased resistance training. Long-term follow-up addresses complications, manages comorbidities, and ensures coordination with other specialties for comprehensive care.

## SUGGESTED READINGS

1. Min K, Beom J, Kim BR, Lee SY, Lee GJ, Lee JH, et al. Clinical practice guideline for postoperative rehabilitation in older patients with hip fractures. Ann Rehabil Med. 2021;45(3):225-59.
2. Sekeitto AR, Sikhauli N, van der Jagt DR, Mokete L, Pietrzak JRT. The management of displaced femoral neck fractures: a narrative review. EFORT Open Rev. 2021;6(2):139-44.
3. Song J, Zhang G, Liang J, Bai C, Dang X, Wang K, et al. Effects of delayed hip replacement on postoperative hip function and quality of life in elderly patients with femoral neck fracture. BMC Musculoskelet Disord. 2020;21:487.
4. Green G, Radha S, Humphreys A. Optimizing outcome once a patient's femoral neck fracture has been operated on. Orthop Trauma. 2020;34(3):174-80.
5. Kale S, Pati B, Srivastava A, Mehta N, Shah V, Chalak A, et al. Evaluating the efficacy of rehabilitation outcomes of the femoral neck system in treating femoral neck fractures: a two-year prospective study. Int J Res Orthop. 2024;10(5):1-4.

# CHAPTER 8

# Complications and Management Strategies

Adarsh Tekumalla, Sandeep Patel, Sachin Yashwant Kale, Arvind J Vatkar, Vishal Kumar

## ■ OVERVIEW OF COMMON COMPLICATIONS ASSOCIATED WITH FEMORAL NECK SYSTEM IMPLANTS

Femoral neck fractures are significant injuries often requiring surgical intervention, typically utilizing femoral neck system (FNS) implants. While these implants offer promising outcomes, they can be associated with complications. Among the most common are nonunion, malunion, avascular necrosis (AVN), and implant-related issues.

Nonunion occurs when the fractured bone fails to heal, leading to persistent pain and functional impairment. Malunion refers to improper alignment of the fracture during healing, resulting in limb-length discrepancy or altered biomechanics. AVN occurs due to compromised blood supply to the femoral head, leading to its deterioration and eventual collapse.

Implant-related complications include implant loosening, breakage, or migration. Loosening can result from inadequate fixation or poor bone quality, leading to instability and pain. Breakage may occur due to excessive stress on the implant, particularly in cases of nonunion or malunion. Migration can lead to altered joint mechanics and increased risk of further complications.

Management of these complications often requires revision surgery, which poses additional risks and challenges. Prevention strategies include careful surgical technique, proper implant selection, and postoperative monitoring. Despite these efforts, complications can still arise, underscoring the importance of thorough preoperative assessment and patient counseling.

## ■ IDENTIFICATION, PREVENTION, AND MANAGEMENT OF COMPLICATIONS DURING THE PERIOPERATIVE PERIOD

Identification, prevention, and management of complications during the perioperative period in orthopedic trauma surgery are paramount for

CHAPTER 8: Complications and Management Strategies

ensuring optimal patient outcomes. Important factors like timing of surgery, patient age, fracture type based on the Pauwels classification, and bone quality significantly influence complication rates.

Timing of surgery plays a crucial role, with early intervention reducing the risk of complications such as infection, delayed union, and nonunion. However, patient factors, including age, must be carefully considered. Older patients often have comorbidities and decreased bone density, necessitating meticulous preoperative assessment and tailored surgical approaches to mitigate complications.

The classification of fractures according to the Pauwels system informs surgical decision-making and predicts the risk of complications. Femoral neck fractures with high Pauwels angle have increased shear force, leading to increased risk of displacement. High-energy fractures with greater displacement are associated with increased complication rates, emphasizing the need for precise reduction and fixation techniques. Hence, it is paramount to have good reduction of fracture fragments, before attempting to fix with FNS.

Bone quality is another critical factor influencing perioperative complications. Poor bone quality, often observed in elderly patients or those with osteoporosis, increases the risk of implant failure and secondary displacement. Strategies such as augmentation techniques and careful implant selection help address these challenges and improve surgical outcomes.

Prevention and early recognition of complications, including infection, implant failure, and neurovascular injury, are integral components of perioperative management. Close monitoring, patient education, and multidisciplinary collaboration facilitate timely intervention and optimize patient recovery.

## ■ STRATEGIES FOR SALVAGE PROCEDURES IN CASE OF IMPLANT FAILURE OR COMPLICATIONS

In orthopedic trauma surgery, encountering implant failure or complications is a challenging yet inevitable aspect of patient care. Salvage procedures are crucial in such scenarios, aiming to rectify the issue while preserving the function and stability of the affected limb. Several strategies can be employed to address implant failure or complications effectively.

Firstly, thorough preoperative planning is paramount. This involves a comprehensive assessment of the patient's medical history, imaging studies, and the specific circumstances surrounding the implant failure or complication. Understanding the underlying cause is essential for devising an appropriate salvage plan.

Secondly, revision surgery may be necessary to replace the malfunctioning implant or address any structural issues. This may involve removing the failed hardware, debriding any infected tissue, and reconstructing the affected area with new implants or alternative fixation techniques.

In some cases, biological augmentation techniques such as bone grafting or biological membranes may be employed to enhance tissue healing and promote implant stability.

Additionally, close postoperative monitoring and rehabilitation are vital components of successful salvage procedures. Regular follow-up visits allow for the early detection of any recurrent issues and enable timely interventions to optimize patient outcomes.

Ultimately, the goal of salvage procedures in orthopedic trauma surgery is to restore function, alleviate pain, and promote patient satisfaction while minimizing the risk of further complications. This requires a multidisciplinary approach, with collaboration between orthopedic surgeons, infectious disease specialists, physical therapists, and other healthcare professionals.

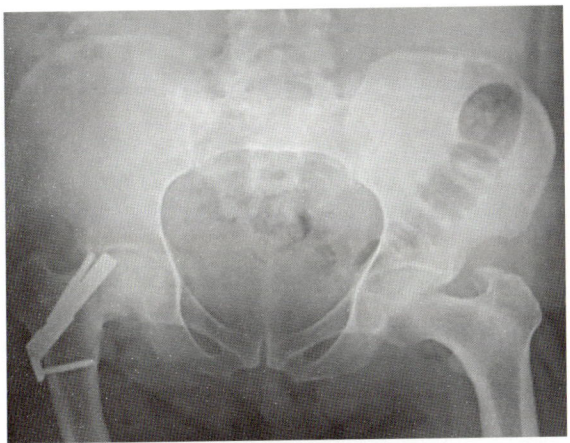

**FIG. 1:** Varus collapse with femoral neck system cut-out.

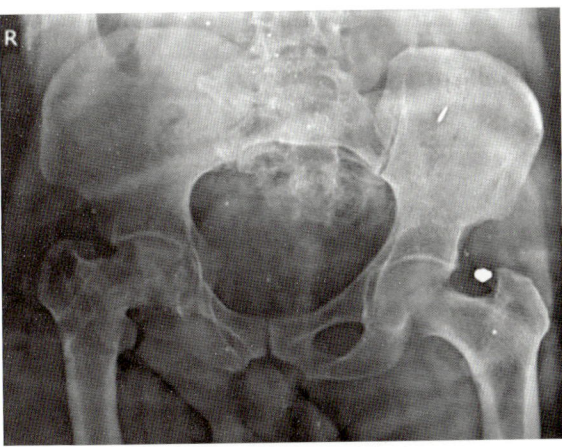

**FIG. 2:** Femoral neck system removed.

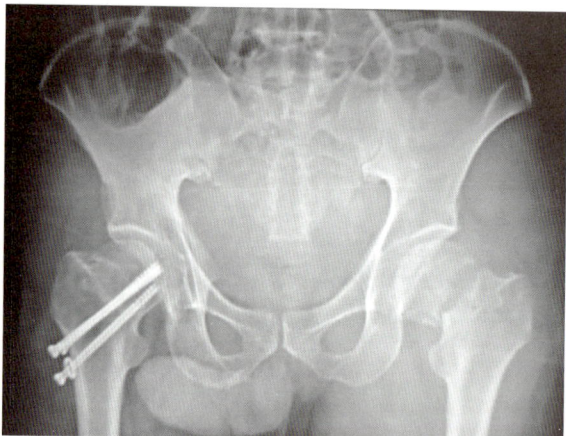

**FIG. 3:** Left-sided subcapital neck femur fracture.

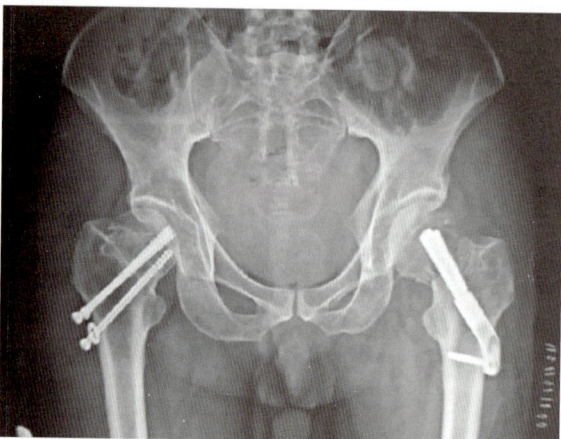

**FIG. 4:** Postoperative X-ray with femoral neck system.

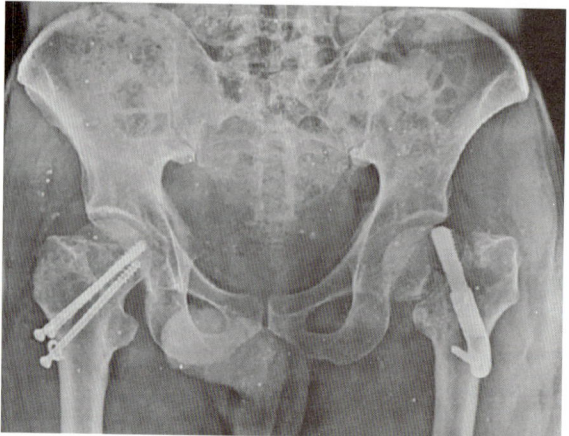

**FIG. 5:** Femoral neck system cut-out with nonunion at 10 months.

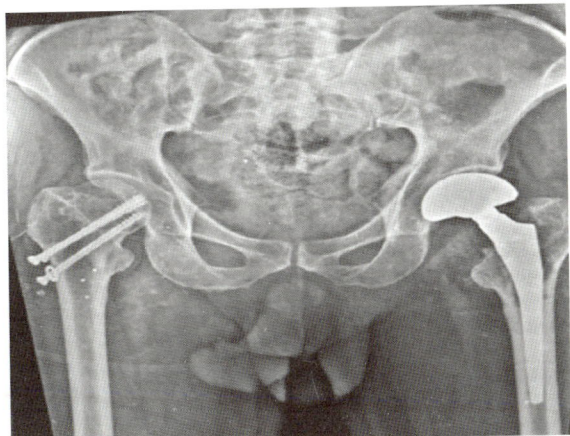

**FIG. 6:** Femoral neck system replaced by bipolar hemiarthroplasty.

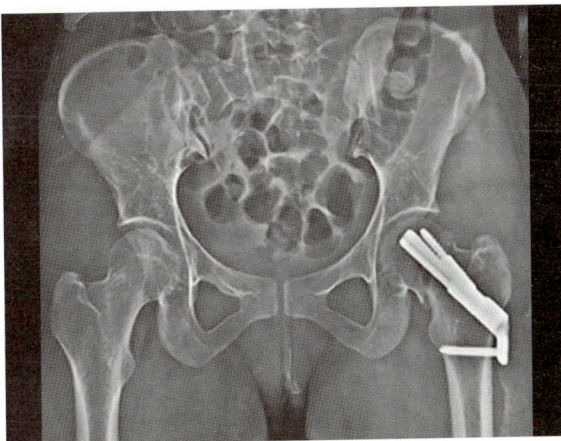

**FIG. 7:** Immediate postoperative X-ray with femoral neck system.

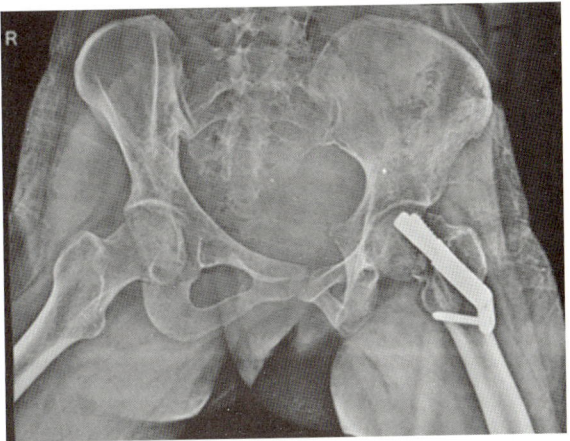

**FIG. 8:** Femoral neck system cut-out at 12 months.

## CHAPTER 8: Complications and Management Strategies

### Summary

A comprehensive understanding of patient-specific factors and meticulous surgical planning are essential for minimizing complications and achieving successful outcomes in orthopedic trauma surgery.

### ■ SUGGESTED READINGS

1. Rajnish RK, Srivastava A, Rathod PM, Haq RU, Aggarwal S, Kumar P, et al. Does the femoral neck system provide better outcomes compared to cannulated screws fixation for the management of femoral neck fracture in young adults? A systematic review of literature and meta-analysis. J Orthop. 2022;32:52-9.
2. Davidson A, Blum S, Harats E, Kachko E, Essa A, Efraty R, et al. Neck of femur fractures treated with the femoral neck system: outcomes of one hundred and two patients and literature review. Int Orthop. 2022;46(9):2105-15.
3. Kale S, Chalak A, Vatkar A, Dey JK, Mehta N, Das S. Limitations and Complications in Treating Femoral Neck Fractures with the Femoral Neck System: A Case Report. J Orthop Case Rep. 2024;14(3):78-82.

# CHAPTER 9

# Outcomes and Clinical Cases

*Pramod Bhor, Shivam Mehra, Sushmit Singh, Sachin Yashwant Kale, Prasad Liladhar Chaudhari*

## ■ REVIEW OF CLINICAL OUTCOMES AND FUNCTIONAL RESULTS FOLLOWING FEMORAL NECK FRACTURE FIXATION

The review of clinical outcomes and functional results following femoral neck fracture fixation is crucial for understanding the effectiveness of various treatment approaches in managing this challenging injury. Several factors influence the outcomes of femoral neck fracture fixation, including patient characteristics, fracture type, surgical technique, implant choice, and postoperative rehabilitation.

Studies assessing clinical outcomes often evaluate parameters such as fracture healing, implant stability, pain relief, functional mobility, and quality of life. Functional outcomes often include measurements of mobility, return to job duties or preinjury degree of activity, and the frequency of problems such as nonunion, avascular necrosis (AVN), and failed implant.

Furthermore, analyzing functional outcomes provides valuable insights into the long-term implications of femoral neck fracture fixation on patients' physical independence and overall well-being. This review synthesizes existing literature to identify trends, disparities, and areas of consensus regarding the efficacy and limitations of different treatment modalities.

By critically evaluating clinical outcomes and functional results, orthopedic surgeons can refine their treatment algorithms, optimize patient selection, and tailor interventions to achieve the best possible outcomes for individuals with femoral neck fractures.

## ■ SUMMARY OF KEY FINDINGS FROM RELEVANT CLINICAL STUDIES AND META-ANALYSES

The summary of key findings from relevant clinical studies and meta-analyses provides a comprehensive overview of the current evidence surrounding femoral neck fracture fixation. Numerous studies have evaluated various fixation techniques, including cannulated screws, dynamic hip screws, and arthroplasty options, to determine their impact on clinical outcomes and functional results.

Meta-analyses have been instrumental in synthesizing data from multiple studies, allowing for a more robust analysis of treatment efficacy and complications. These analyses have highlighted important considerations such as the risk of nonunion, AVN, and implant-related complications associated with different fixation methods.

Furthermore, studies have explored factors influencing treatment outcomes, including patient age, fracture displacement, and surgical timing. Understanding these factors is crucial for tailoring treatment approaches to individual patient needs and optimizing outcomes.

Overall, the summary of key findings underscores the importance of evidence-based decision-making in femoral neck fracture management. By synthesizing data from clinical studies and meta-analyses, clinicians can make informed decisions regarding treatment strategies, ultimately improving patient care and long-term outcomes.

## ■ DISCUSSION ON THE EVIDENCE-BASED APPROACH TO DECISION-MAKING IN FEMORAL NECK FRACTURE MANAGEMENT

Discussion on the evidence-based approach to decision-making in femoral neck fracture management revolves around synthesizing findings from clinical studies and meta-analyses to inform treatment strategies. By scrutinizing the outcomes and functional results following femoral neck fracture fixation, clinicians can refine their approach to patient care.

An evidence-based approach entails weighing the efficacy, safety, and long-term implications of various treatment options. For instance, comparing the outcomes of internal fixation versus arthroplasty in different patient populations can guide surgeons in selecting the most suitable intervention based on factors such as age, comorbidities, and fracture characteristics.

Furthermore, understanding the nuances of surgical techniques, implant choices, and postoperative rehabilitation protocols is crucial for optimizing patient outcomes. By critically evaluating the evidence, clinicians can tailor their management approach to individual patient needs while minimizing the risk of complications and maximizing functional recovery.

Moreover, ongoing research and advancements in surgical technology continue to shape the landscape of femoral neck fracture management. Integrating emerging evidence into clinical practice ensures that patients receive the most effective and evidence-based care, ultimately improving outcomes and enhancing quality of life.

# CHAPTER 9: Outcomes and Clinical Cases

## CASELETS

### Case 1

A 20-year-old male had a transcervical neck femur fracture (**Figs. 1 to 3**).

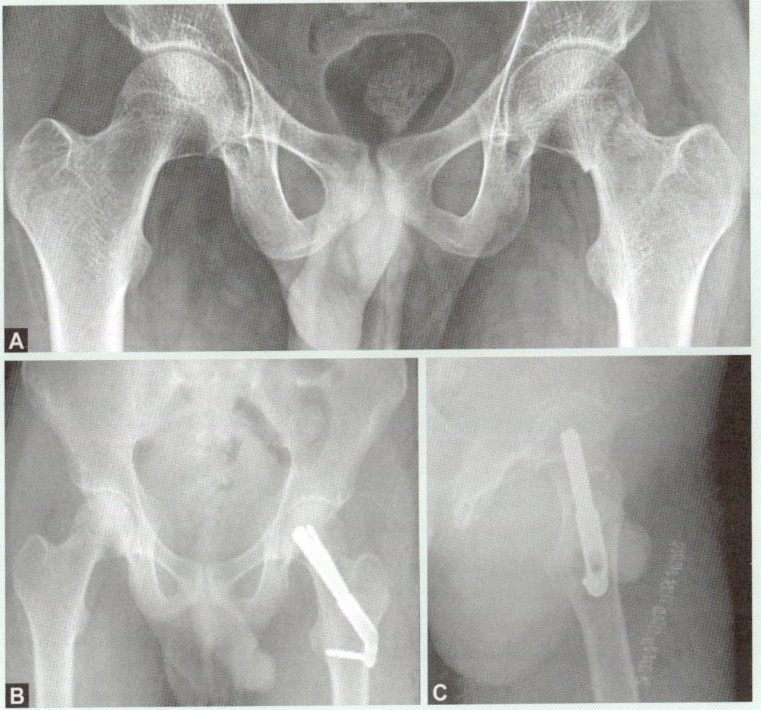

**FIGS. 1A TO C:** Immediate postoperative X-rays.

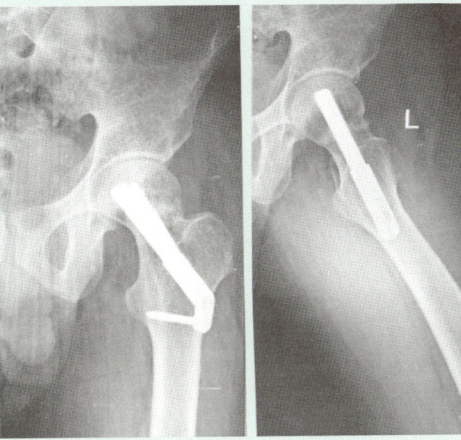

**FIG. 2:** X-rays showing union.

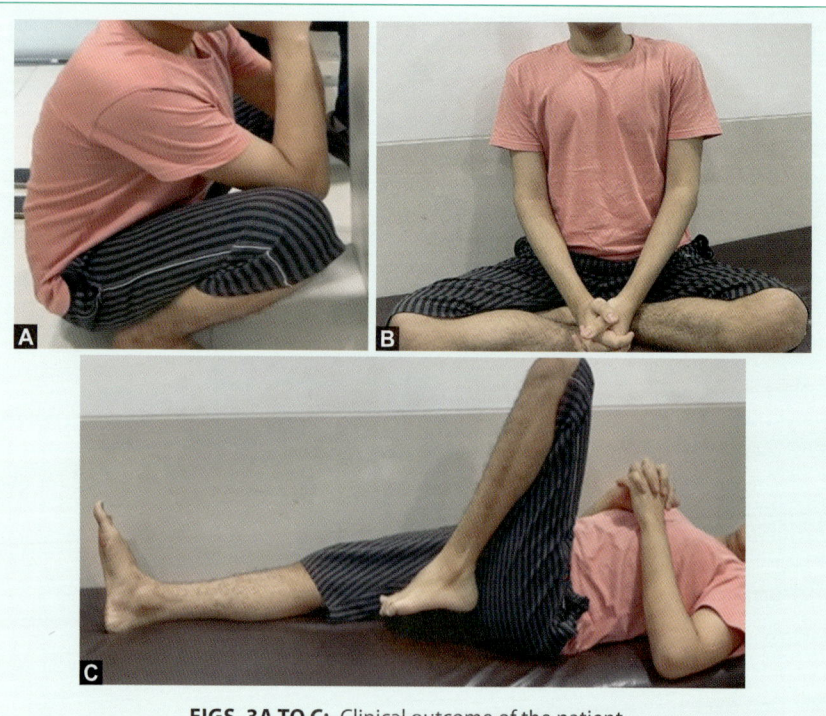

**FIGS. 3A TO C:** Clinical outcome of the patient.

## Case 2

A 28-year-old male had a displaced basicervical neck femur fracture (**Figs. 4 and 5**).

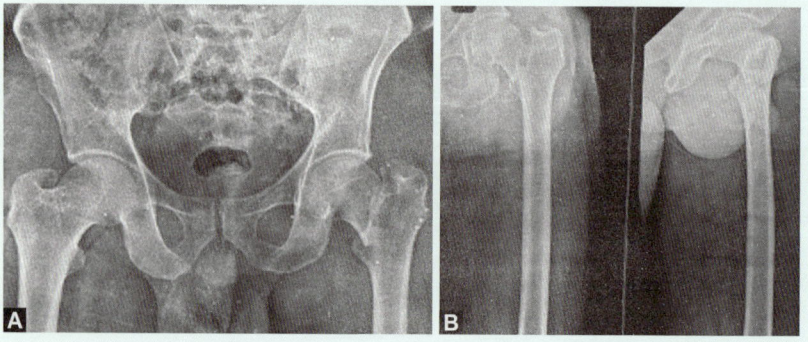

**FIGS. 4A TO E:** *Continued*

# CHAPTER 9: Outcomes and Clinical Cases

*Continued*

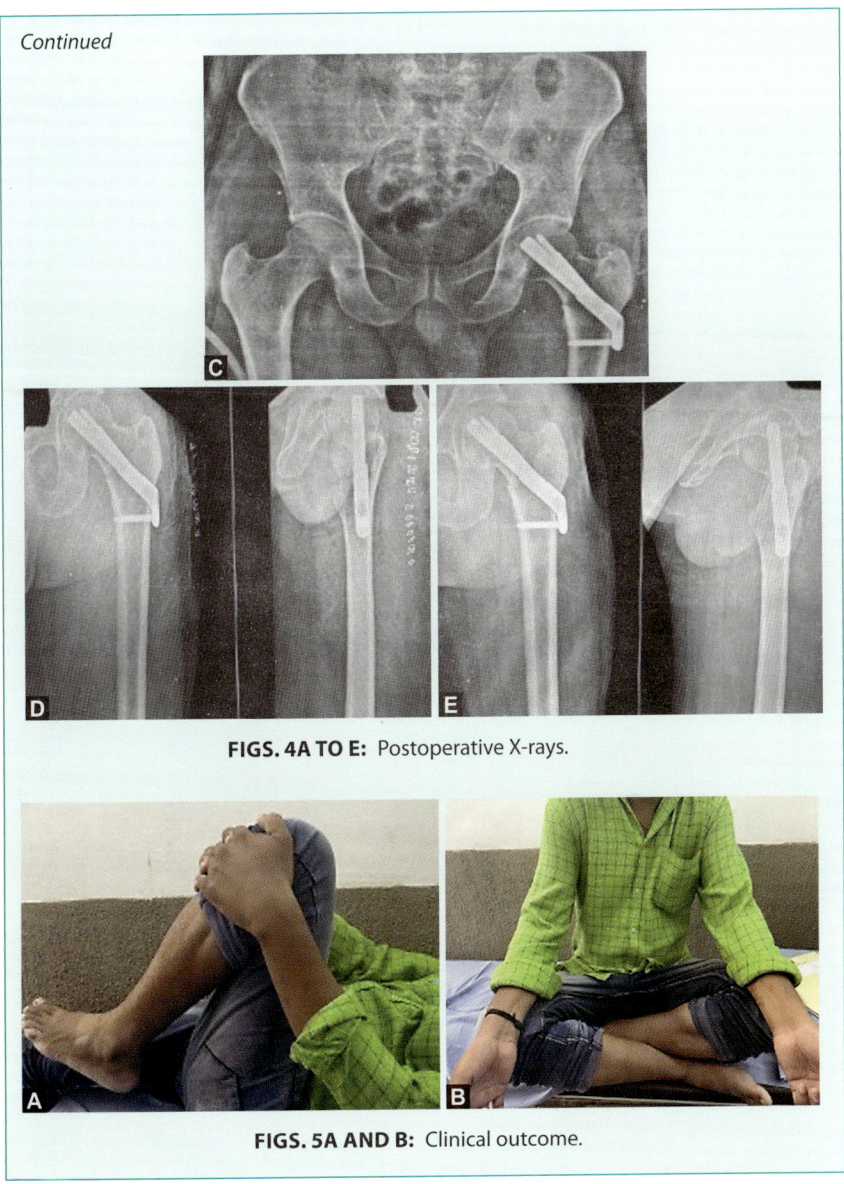

**FIGS. 4A TO E:** Postoperative X-rays.

**FIGS. 5A AND B:** Clinical outcome.

## Case 3

An 18-year-old female had left subcapital neck femur fracture **(Figs. 6 and 7)**.

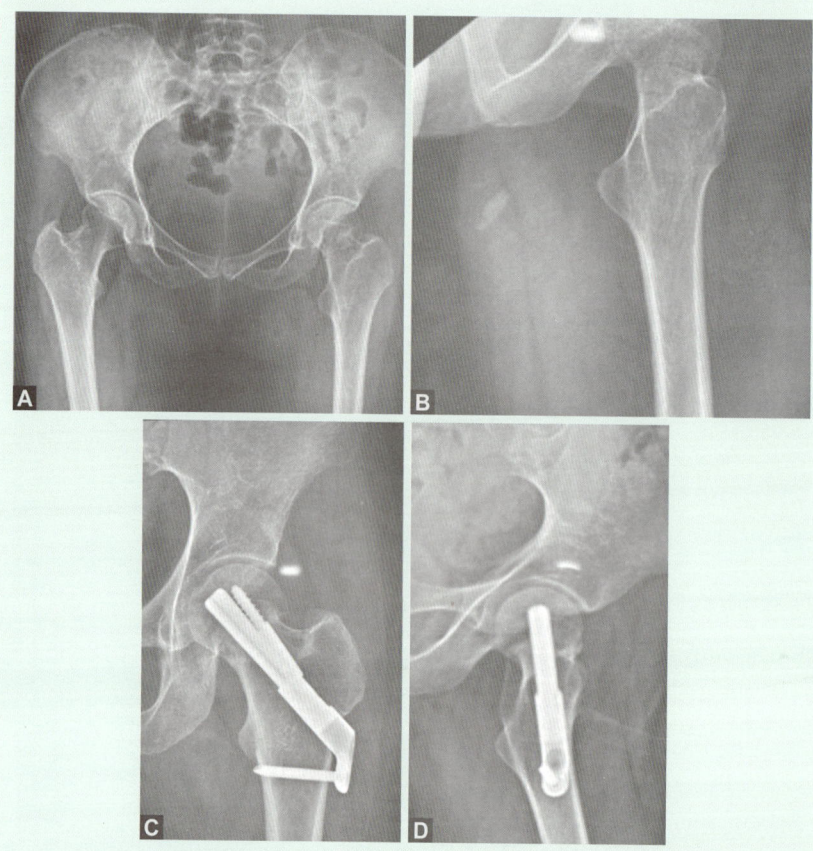

**FIGS. 6A TO D:** X-rays showing union.

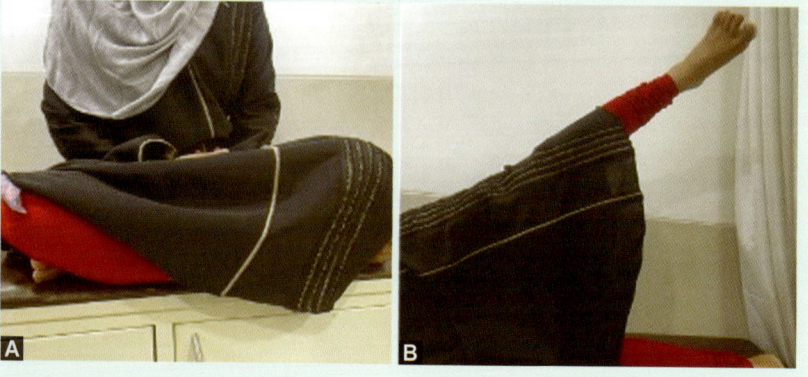

**FIGS. 7A TO D:** *Continued*

Continued

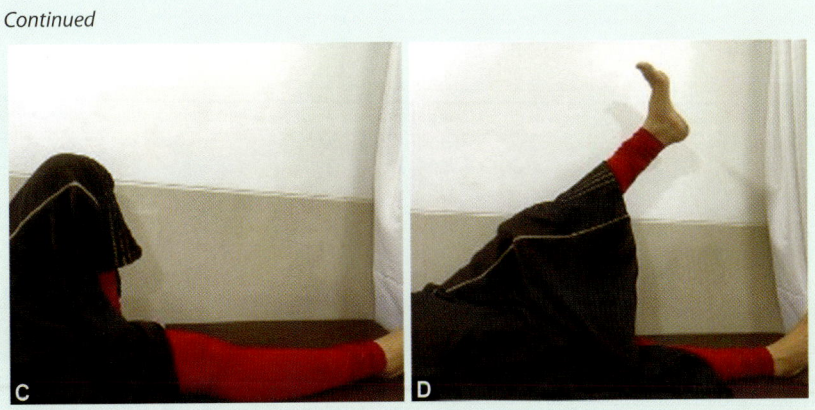

**FIGS. 7A TO D:** Clinical outcome.

## Case 4

A 34-year-old patient had displaced right transcervical neck femur fracture (**Figs. 8 and 9**).

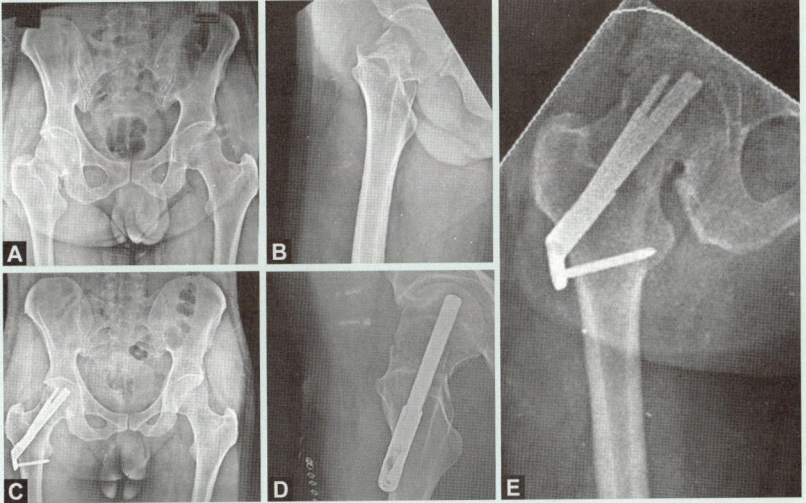

**FIGS. 8A TO E:** X-ray photograph showing: (A) Preoperative AP view—right neck of femur fracture; (B) Preoperative lateral view—right hip-neck of femur fracture; (C) Postoperative AP view—FNS fixation; (D) Postoperative lateral view—FNS fixation; (E) 3 months postoperative view of FNS fixation.

**44** CHAPTER 9: Outcomes and Clinical Cases

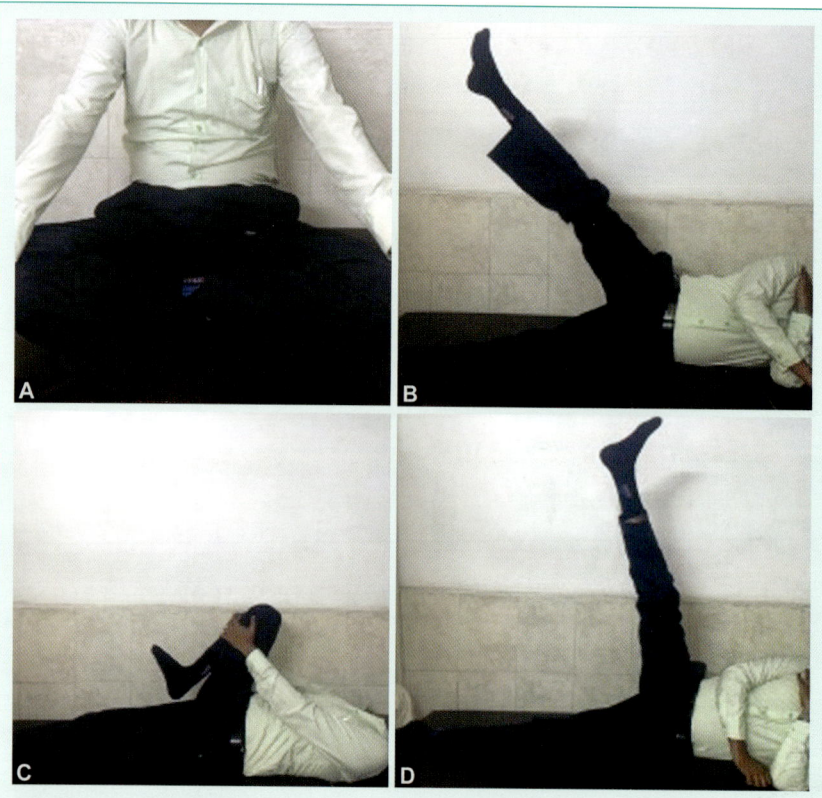

**FIGS. 9A TO D:** Clinical outcome of the patient.

## Case 5

A 26-year-old male had right subcapital neck femur fracture **(Figs. 10 and 11)**.

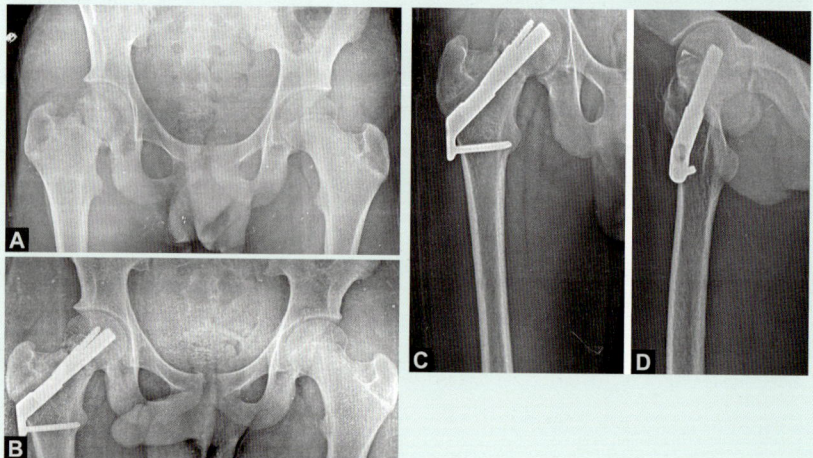

**FIGS. 10A TO D:** X-ray photos showing initial fracture (A), immediate postoperative X-ray (B), and follow-up X-ray of hip AP and lateral view (C and D).

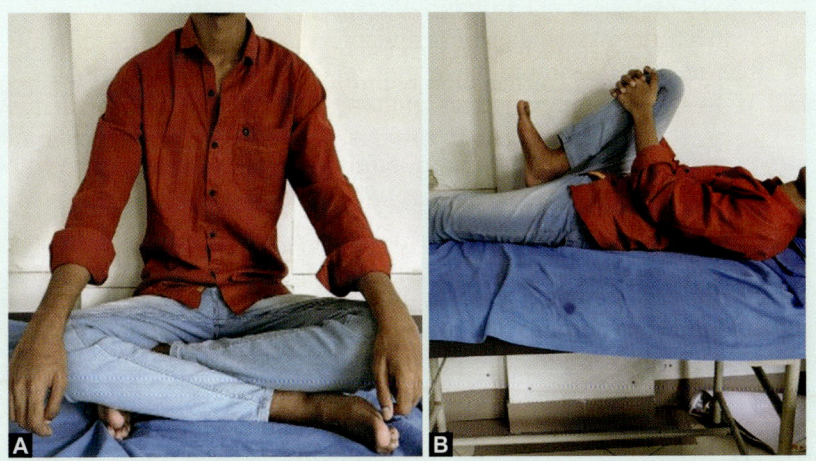

**FIGS. 11A AND B:** Clinical outcome.

## Case 6

A 39-year-old had impacted left transcervical neck femur fractures (**Figs. 12 and 13**).

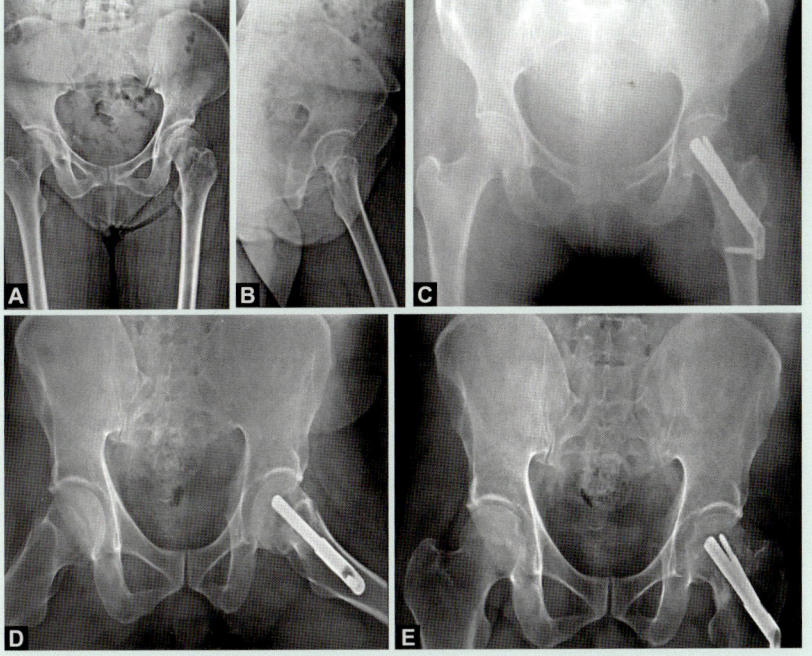

**FIGS. 12A TO E:** X-rays showing union.

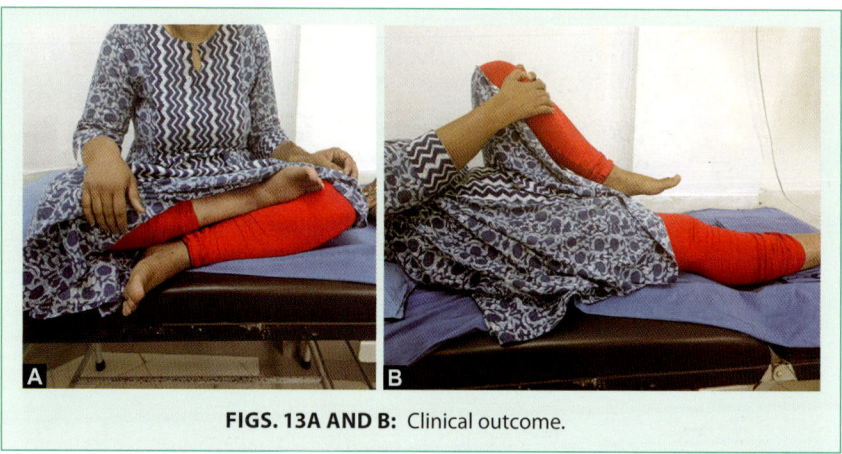

**FIGS. 13A AND B:** Clinical outcome.

## Summary

Reviewing clinical outcomes and functional results after femoral neck fracture fixation is essential for evaluating treatment effectiveness, influenced by patient characteristics, fracture type, surgical technique, implant choice, and rehabilitation. Studies assess parameters like fracture healing, implant stability, pain relief, mobility, and quality of life. Meta-analyses synthesize data on complications such as nonunion, AVN, and implant-related issues, guiding evidence-based decision-making for personalized patient care and optimal outcomes.

## ■ SUGGESTED READINGS

1. Davidson A, Blum S, Harats E, Kachko E, Essa A, Efraty R, et al. Neck of femur fractures treated with the femoral neck system: outcomes of one hundred and two patients and literature review. Int Orthop. 2022;46(9):2105-15.
2. Stassen RC, Jeuken RM, Boonen B, Meesters B, de Loos ER, van Vugt R. First clinical results of 1-year follow-up of the femoral neck system for internal fixation of femoral neck fractures. Arch Orthop Trauma Surg. 2022;142(12):3755-63.
3. Hu H, Cheng J, Feng M, Gao Z, Wu J, Lu S. Clinical outcome of femoral neck system versus cannulated compression screws for fixation of femoral neck fracture in younger patients. J Orthop Surg Res. 2021;16(1):370.

# 10 CHAPTER

# Future Perspectives and Innovations

Ajit Chalak, Gaurav Kanade, Sachin Yashwant Kale, Nindiya Kapoor Mehra, Smruti Sachin Kale, Sandeep N Deore

## ■ EMERGING TRENDS AND ADVANCEMENTS IN FEMORAL NECK SYSTEM IMPLANTS

According to the nature of fracture, the condition of the bone, and age of the patient, surgical therapies for neck of femur (NOF) fractures include arthroplasty or internal fixation. Currently, the most often utilized implants are cannulated cancellous screws (CCS), dynamic hip screws (DHS), and femoral neck system (FNS). FNS, the most recently designed implant, integrates compression as well as antirotation properties, demonstrating good biomechanical and clinical results when compared to previous femoral neck fracture (FNF) treatment implant options.

Recent advances employ orthopedic surgery robot positioning systems for precise internal fixation of FNS. The recent studies have shown that the robot can improvise on the accuracy of placement of the guide needle during treatment of FNFs with cannulated screws and shorten the time of operative procedure as well as reduce injury due to surgery and X-ray compared with traditional technique that is non-navigated. The conventional placing of the FNS is dependent on the surgeons' experience. Due to human errors, incorrect positioning can cause postoperative complications. To minimize these risks, orthopedic robots are a recent advancement in the placement of FNS implants.

## ■ PREDICTIONS FOR THE FUTURE DIRECTION OF RESEARCH AND TECHNOLOGY IN THIS FIELD

Future direction of research in this field might involve the role of artificial intelligence (AI) and 3D bioprinting to design patient specific implants that are tailor-made depending upon factors like fracture pattern, osteoporosis, duration of surgery, comorbidities, and prior surgery. Patient-specific implants will ensure reduced rate of nonunion as well as improved osteosynthesis. Another powerful role of AI will be in the diagnosis of hip fractures together with the use of robot navigation systems for precise placement of the implant.

CHAPTER 10: Future Perspectives and Innovations

## ■ RECOMMENDATIONS FOR CONTINUED PROFESSIONAL DEVELOPMENT AND STAYING ABREAST OF NEW DEVELOPMENTS

Continued professional development (CPD) is essential for orthopedic surgeons and healthcare professionals specializing in femoral neck fractures to maintain their skills, improve outcomes, and stay updated with the latest advancements. Here are key recommendations for effective CPD and staying abreast of new developments in the management of femoral neck fractures:

1. *Engage in Specialized Training and Education*: Participating in orthopedic-specific workshops and conferences provides hands-on experience and exposure to the latest research and surgical techniques. Pursuing certifications in orthopedic trauma or geriatric orthopedics ensures a deep understanding of femoral neck fractures, especially in the elderly, who are most affected by this injury.
2. *Utilize Online Learning Resources*: Online platforms offer numerous courses and webinars focused on femoral neck fractures, covering topics from surgical techniques to rehabilitation. These resources provide flexibility to learn at one's own pace. Subscribing to Related Research journals keeps professionals updated on the latest studies, clinical trials, and treatment guidelines.
3. *Participate in Professional Organizations*: Joining professional societies and engaging within these organizations focuses learning on femoral neck fractures, offering targeted education and collaboration opportunities.
4. *Collaborate and Research*: Engaging with colleagues through case discussions and peer reviews enhances knowledge. Active involvement in clinical research on femoral neck fractures helps in understanding advancements and contributes to the medical community.
5. *Stay Updated with Technological Advances*: Regularly updating knowledge on new surgical techniques, implants, and diagnostic tools is crucial. Simulation training for new procedures ensures proficiency without patient risk.

## Summary

Commitment to CPD through specialized training, leveraging online resources, active participation in professional organizations, collaboration, research, and staying updated with technological advancements ensures orthopedic professionals remain at the forefront of femoral neck fracture management. This ongoing learning and adaptation are key to improving patient outcomes and advancing the field of orthopedics.

# CHAPTER 11

# Conclusion: Summary and Key Takeaways

*Sachin Yashwant Kale, Aditya Gupta, Vishal Kumar, Arvind J Vatkar*

Because of the significant risk of nonunion and avascular necrosis (AVN), NOF fracture is still referred to as a "unsolved fracture". The therapy varies according to the age and fracture type. The surgical treatment of elderly individuals is straightforward, often requiring one of many types of arthroplasty surgeries. In young patients, it is based on Pauwels' categorization and the anatomical site of the fracture. Type I Pauwels' fractures are treated by partially threaded cannulated screws (PTCS) used in either an inverted triangular configuration or quadrangular configuration (for communition). BDSF (biplane double-supported screw fixation) creates a two-point support and biplane positioning of screws; it improves the stability of the fracture neck femur and can enhance constant stability during various patient activities. Type II and type III Pauwels' fracture in young patients are managed with sliding hip screw (SHS) or FNS **(Figs. 1A and B)**. FNS offers a reduced complication percentage, faster union, and superior clinical results. The decreased complication rates

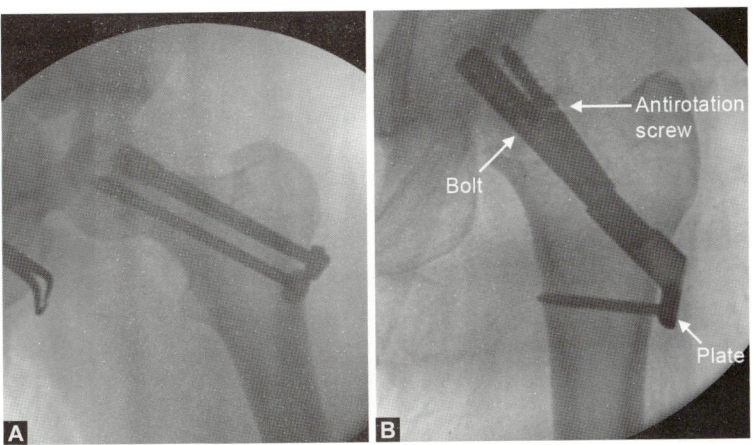

**FIGS. 1A AND B:** Femoral neck system (FNS) and partially threaded cannulated screws (PTCS) in inverted triangle configuration.

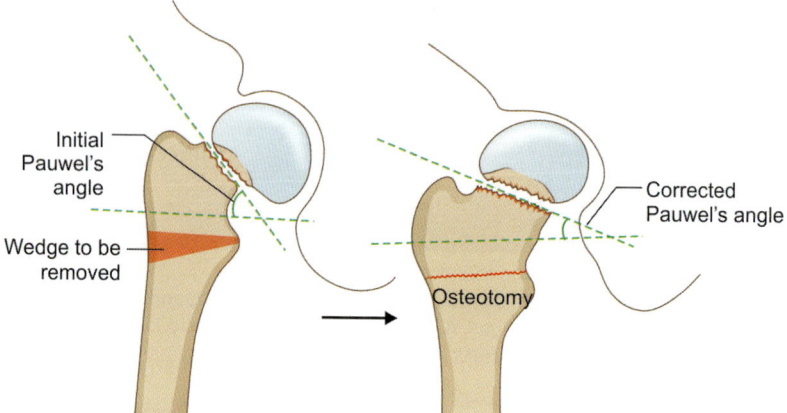

**FIG. 2:** Valgus closing wedge osteotomy at the intertrochanteric region, converts shear forces at the fracture site to compression forces by decreasing Pauwel's angle.

associated with healing of wounds, internal fixation collapse with screw cut-out with loosening, loss of reduction, nonunion, and AVN can be attributed to the FNS design. FNS and DHS showed comparable biomechanics and were much stronger than CCS fixation.

No matter which treatment pattern is used the reduction of the femoral alignment and neck remains imperative to the prognosis and decreasing the chances of AVN and osteonecrosis. Garden alignment index and Lowell S curves indicate good reduction intraoperatively. Nonunion is a challenging problem after fracture femoral neck in young adults. It can be managed with intertrochanteric valgus osteotomy **(Fig. 2)**, vascularized bone grafting, or arthroplasty procedures. Use of robotic systems can ensure optimal placement of the guidewire further reducing the rate of complications like implant failure.

The femoral neck system (FNS) offers several advantages over other fixation devices based on clinical evidence and data:

- *Reduced operative time*: FNS provides angular and rotational stability, facilitating insertion through reduced incision size, potentially leading to reduced operative time.
- *Economic value*: FNS is associated with reduced rates of reoperation, potentially leading to cost savings for the healthcare system.
- *Improved clinical outcomes*: Studies have shown that FNS is associated with lower rates of overall complications, nonunion, femoral neck shortening, and intraoperative fluoroscopies compared to other fixation devices.
- *Enhanced stability*: FNS offers at least 150% more rotational stability and at least 100% more resistance to varus collapse compared to other fixation devices.

- *Reduced invasiveness*: FNS is designed to minimize implant footprint on the bone, reduce incision size, and reduce protrusion, potentially leading to reduced blood loss and length of stay.
- *Faster recovery*: FNS use has been associated with faster recovery and shorter hospitalization time compared to other treatment options for femoral neck fractures.

These factors collectively contribute to the superior performance of the FNS compared to other fixation devices, as supported by clinical studies and data.

## SUGGESTED READINGS

1. Davidovitch RI, Jordan CJ, Egol KA, Vrahas MS. Challenges in the treatment of femoral neck fractures in the nonelderly adult. J Trauma. 2010;68:236-42.
2. Patel S, Kumar V, Baburaj V, Dhillon MS. The use of the femoral neck system (FNS) leads to better outcomes in the surgical management of femoral neck fractures in adults compared to fixation with cannulated screws: A systematic review and meta-analysis. Eur J Orthop Surg Traumatol. 2023;33(5):2101-29.
3. Stoffel K, Zderic I, Gras F, Sommer C, Eberli U, Mueller D, et al. Biomechanical evaluation of the femoral neck system in unstable Pauwels III femoral neck Fractures: A comparison with the dynamic hip screw and cannulated screws. J Orthop Trauma. 2017;31:131-7.
4. Keller CS, Laros GS. Indications for open reduction of femoral neck fractures. Clin Orthop Relat Res. 1980;(152):131-7.

# Publications

1. Kale S, Mishra R, Singh S, Chalak A, Vatkar A, Ghodke R, et al. A prospective study to analyze the functional outcome of the femoral neck system in femoral neck fractures. MGM J Med Sci. 2023;10(3):409-14.
2. Patel S, Kumar V, Baburaj V, Dhillon MS. The use of the femoral neck system (FNS) leads to better outcomes in the surgical management of femoral neck fractures in adults compared to fixation with cannulated screws: A systematic review and meta-analysis. Eur J Orthop Surg Traumatol. 2023;33(5):2101-9.
3. Vatkar A, Kale S, Kanade G, Godke A, Dey JK, Godke R, et al. Comparing the Efficiency of the Femoral Neck System and the Cannulated Compression Screw in Treating Femoral Neck Fractures in Patients Who Are Young and Middle-aged Indian Population. J Clin Orthop. 2023;8(2):16-20.
4. Kale S, Chalak A, Vatkar A, Dey JK, Mehta N, Das S. Limitations and Complications in Treating Femoral Neck Fractures with the Femoral Neck System: A Case Report. J Orthop Case Rep. 2024;14(3):78-82.
5. Kale S, Pati B, Srivastava A, Mehta N, Shah V, Chalak A, et al. Evaluating the efficacy of rehabilitation outcomes of the femoral neck system in treating femoral neck fractures: a two-year prospective study. Int J Res Orthop. 2024;10(5):1-4.

# Index

Page numbers followed by *f* refer to figure.

## A

Advanced trauma life support 18, 19
Ambulation training 28
Artificial intelligence 47
Avascular necrosis 1, 7, 11, 31, 37, 49

## B

Basicervical neck femur fracture 40
Biomechanical principles 8
Bipolar hemiarthroplasty 35*f*
Blood
   circulation 28
   supply 78*f*
Bone quality 32

## C

Calcar femorale 7
   preservation of 7
Cannulated cancellous screws 47
Cannulated compression screws 13, 16
Cannulated screw 12, 13
   systems 12
C-arm guidance 24
Casting 11
Central guidewire 24
Computed tomography scans 19

## D

Deep vein thrombosis 5
Dynamic hip screws 11, 12, 14, 16, 47

## E

Early fixation techniques 11

## F

Femoral bone, lateral compartments
   of 23*f*
Femoral capsule 8
Femoral head 24*f*
   avascular necrosis of 5
Femoral neck 7, 9, 24, 24*f*
   anatomy of 7
   biomechanics of 7
   fracture 1, 3-5, 8, 18, 31
      classification of 1, 3*f*
      fixation 22, 37
      Garden classification of 3*f*
      management 38
      treatment 11, 14
   intricate vascular supply 8
   system 12, 14, 15, 16*f*, 17*f*, 18, 25*f*, 34*f*,
      35*f*, 47, 49*f*, 50
      cut-out 33, 34*f*, 35*f*
      implants 11, 15, 31, 47
      removed 33*f*
Femur fracture 43*f*
   hip neck of 43*f*
   nature of 1, 7
Femur, nature of 18, 47
Fracture 3*f*, 44*f*
   displacement 20
   nature of 47
   site 24

## G

Garden alignment 50
Garden classification 3*f*
   system 1
Garden screw 11, 12*f*
Greater trochanter 23*f*

# Index

## H

Hip
  fractures 3
  joint, capsule of 8

## I

Implant
  failure 32
  proper placement of 27
Internal fixation 11

## L

Lateral circumflex femoral artery 7

## M

Magnetic resonance imaging 19
Medial circumflex femoral artery 7
Mobilization, early 28
Modern implants, concept of 13
Motion exercises, range of 28

## N

Neck femur fracture 42-45

## O

Orthopedic traction table 22
Orthopedic trauma surgery 32, 36
Osteoporotic bone 12, 20

## P

Pain management 28
Partially threaded cannulated screws 49$f$
Pauwels' angle 50$f$
Pauwels' categorization 49
Pauwels' classification 1
  method 9
Pauwels' fracture 49
Pins 11
Proximal femur, blood supply of 8$f$
Pulmonary embolism 5

## Q

Quality-adjusted life years 4

## R

Reaming 25$f$
Rehabilitation protocols 28
Respiratory health 28

## S

Salvage procedures 32
Screws 11
Sliding hip screw 12, 49
Smith–Peterson nail 12, 12$f$
Subcapital neck femur fracture 34$f$

## T

Threaded cannulated screws 49
Traction 11
Transcervical neck femur fracture 39

## V

Valgus closing wedge osteotomy 50$f$
Various fixation methods, comparative analysis of 13
Varus collapse 33$f$

## W

Watson–Jones approach 22
Weight-bearing progression 28

## X

X-rays 19, 27$f$, 39$f$, 41$f$, 42$f$, 45$f$